WHOLE PERSON CARING

An Interprofessional Model for Healing and Wellness

Lucia Thornton, MSN, RN, AHN-BC

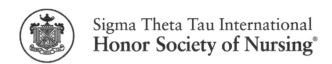

Sigma Theta Tau International
Honor Society of Nursing®

The Honor Society of Nursing, Sigma Theta Tau International (STTI) is a nonprofit organization whose mission is to support the learning, knowledge, and professional development of nurses committed to making a difference in health worldwide. Founded in 1922, STTI has 130,000 members in 86 countries. Members include practicing nurses, instructors, researchers, policymakers, entrepreneurs, and others. STTI's 488 chapters are located at 668 institutions of higher education throughout Australia, Botswana, Brazil, Canada, Colombia, Ghana, Hong Kong, Japan, Kenya, Malawi, Mexico, the Netherlands, Pakistan, Portugal, Singapore, South Africa, South Korea, Swaziland, Sweden, Taiwan, Tanzania, United Kingdom, United States, and Wales. More information about STTI can be found online at www.nursingsociety.org.

Sigma Theta Tau International
550 West North Street
Indianapolis, IN, USA 46202

To order additional books, buy in bulk, or order for corporate use, contact Nursing Knowledge International at 888.NKI.4YOU (888.654.4968/US and Canada) or +1.317.634.8171 (outside US and Canada).

To request a review copy for course adoption, e-mail solutions@nursingknowledge.org or call 888.NKI.4YOU (888.654.4968/US and Canada) or +1.317.634.8171 (outside US and Canada).

To request author information, or for speaker or other media requests, contact Marketing, Honor Society of Nursing, Sigma Theta Tau International at 888.634.7575 (US and Canada) or +1.317.634.8171 (outside US and Canada).

ISBN: 9781937554996
EPUB ISBN: 9781938835001
PDF ISBN: 9781938835018
MOBI ISBN: 9781938835025

Library of Congress Cataloging-in-Publication data

Thornton, Lucia, 1952-
    Whole person care : an Interprofessional model for healing and wellness / Lucia Thornton.
        p. ; cm.
    Includes bibliographical references.
    ISBN 978-1-937554-99-6 (book : alk. paper) -- ISBN 978-1-938835-00-1 (EPUB) -- ISBN 978-1-938835-01-8 (PDF) -- ISBN 978-1-938835-02-5 (MOBI)
    I. Sigma Theta Tau International. II. Title.
    [DNLM: 1. Holistic Nursing--standards. 2. Holistic Health--standards. 3. Models, Nursing. 4. Nursing Staff--standards. 5. Organizational Culture. WY 86.5]
    RT41
    610.73--dc23
                                2013014474

First Printing, 2013

Publisher: Renee Wilmeth
Acquisitions Editor: Emily Hatch
Editorial Coordinator: Paula Jeffers
Cover Designer: Rebecca Batchelor
Interior Design/Page Layout: Rebecca Batchelor

Principal Book Editor: Carla Hall
Development and Project Editor: Kate Shoup
Copy Editor: Erin Geile
Proofreader: Jennifer Lynn
Indexer: Joy Dean Lee
Production Coordinator: Andrew Kimmel

Dedication

To my son David, whose light shone brightly for too short a time on this earth; to my daughter Christy, whose light continues to shine brightly; and to my husband Rod, whose wonderful support has enabled me to pursue this work.

Acknowledgments

I am ever grateful for those people who have directly and indirectly contributed to the ideas and concepts expressed in this book. I have had the opportunity to be influenced by and learn from pioneers in holistic medicine. The founders of the American Holistic Medical Association—Gladys McGarey, Evarts Loomis, and Norm Shealy—and a pioneer in biofeedback—Elmer Green—have been wonderful teachers and always met and continue to meet my inquiries with open hearts and open minds. They have inspired me and helped me understand some of the dynamics involved in healing and wellness. I am ever grateful for their insights, their wisdom, and their inspiration throughout the years. They have been wonderful friends, mentors, and teachers.

I am most grateful to Martha Rogers for her brilliant, innovative, and futuristic thinking. Her theory of unitary human beings has influenced many of the concepts of whole-person caring and has guided nursing into the 21st century. Martha was a wonderful advisor and mentor whose caring and compassionate way of being was ever-present. While she is missed, her presence continues to be felt in this work and the work of so many of her students.

Jean Watson has been an important influence in promoting a caring and healing paradigm. Jean's work in developing and promoting her caring science has helped restore caring and healing as a central focus and mission of nursing. Her work in promoting the role of spirituality in nursing and being the first to talk about the soul in nursing literature make Jean a trailblazer in bringing healing back into nursing. The concepts of caring and healing are foundational to the model of whole-person caring and much gratitude is extended to Jean for her undying efforts in developing and nurturing these concepts throughout her life.

While many theorists, practitioners, and scientists will be mentioned within the context of this book, there are many other people who have influenced my thinking and have been great teachers for me throughout the years. Their writings and teachings have opened my mind and expanded my view of the universe. While I have had the opportunity to study with and learn from many of these teachers in person, others I have learned from through the wisdom in their writings. I am particularly grateful to Pierre Teilhard de Chardin and Paramahansa Yogananda, whose teachings and wisdom have had a major influence in my life, my work, and my view of the universe.

I am also very grateful to those friends, past and present, who inspire me, fill my soul with joy, expand my horizons, and continually increase my understanding of healing. Much gratitude goes to Judith Lau, Anne Dupontavice, Nancy Hinds, Richard Moss, Harrison Madden, Harry Owens, Celia Coates, Jack and Judy Stucki, Bernice Hill, Bram Sheafor, Gilah Hirsch, Bob and Ann Nunley, Herb and Wanda Blumenthal, Bernie Williams, Jim Oschman, Leonard Wisneski, Dan Benor, Rebecca Good, Cay Randall-May, Scott Walker and all of my Council Grove family and Council for Healing friends and colleagues.

Two people were key in the direct development of the model of whole-person caring. Jeanie Gold and Darlene Pedersen contributed immensely to the development of the model. Jeanie Gold and I spent countless hours envisioning and imagining a system of health care that could facilitate healing and wellness. Jeanie's contributions to the model and the development of early educational programs were inspiring, essential, and foundational. Bringing the model to life and my befriending of technology could not have happened without Darlene Pedersen, whose computer expertise and knowledge of all things technological helped create some of the animated PowerPoint presentations and computer setups for our educational programs.

The model of whole-person caring was brought to life in the workplace through the efforts of a remarkable group of nurses. Marilyn Watkins, a nurse manager, and Diane Sheldon, a director of clinical services, understood the importance of integrating concepts of healing and wellness into the heart of their hospital. These two leaders sustained the vision and supported the efforts of a core group of nurses who helped implement the needed changes on the front lines of patient care. This core group of nurses became models of wellness and created a caring-healing presence that transformed their workplace. Kathy Mahannah, Laurie Wilson, Sherry Wildey, and Sue Young were nurses in the core group whose perseverance and commitment helped transform their hospital into a healing environment.

Much appreciation is extended to those who contributed to the content of this book. First, I must thank my daughter, Christy, who contributed her expertise in the area of nutrition and exercise in writing the major portion of Chapter 8. I so admire all that she manifests in this world and feel blessed to have her in my life. Special appreciation is also extended to my son, David, and to the "collective knowingness of this topic" for their contributions and information. David continues to be a source of inspiration in my life and a bridge to the infinite nature of existence.

I would like to thank those who gave their permission to reproduce some of their work in this book. Special thanks to Ka-Kit Hui, MD, medical director for the UCLA Center for East-West Medicine, for permission to reproduce the information in the "Five Essential Acupressure Points" brochure that he developed. Permission to use the Jin Shin Jyutsu charts and information for self-care practices was generously provided by David Burmeister, the director of Jin Shin Jyutsu, Inc., and the hand and foot reflexology charts were graciously provided by Melvin Powers Publishing.

Finally, I would like to thank the publishing team at Sigma Theta Tau International for guiding and orchestrating the development, editing, and layout of this book. Special thanks goes to Emily Hatch, acquisitions editor, who held my hand and answered my seemingly endless questions with extreme patience and goodwill; Erin Geile, copy editor, whose attention to detail and editing prowess is extraordinary; and Kate Shoup, development and project editor, whose ability to see the whole picture and to organize and edit content is quite exceptional. Also, deep appreciation is extended to those working behind the scenes and exquisitely managing all the other aspects of publishing and marketing: Carla Hall, principal book editor; Renee Wilmeth, publisher; Andrew Kimmel, production coordinator; Paula Jeffers, editorial coordinator; Rebecca Batchelor, cover and book designer; Jennifer Lynn, proofreader; and Joy Dean Lee, indexer. Many thanks to a wonderful team!

About the Author

Lucia Thornton, MSN, RN, AHN-BC

Lucia Thornton has been involved in nursing, holistic healing, and health care for more than 35 years. She has held clinical, managerial, and administrative positions in various organizations and settings including emergency and trauma, intensive care, education, and research and development. She helped develop one of the first in-patient hospice homes in the country. She was instrumental in creating the process of board certification for holistic nursing in the United States and served as the first executive director of the American Holistic Nurses Certification Corporation. She established and directed The Visions in Healthcare Council and The Institute of Health and Well-Being to foster an awareness of health and healing in her community. Her teaching experience includes teaching undergraduate and graduate nursing students at California State University in Fresno and offering programs on holistic nursing across the country.

For the past 10 years, she has been involved with developing seminars for hospitals and communities that focus on staff development and creating healing environments. She uses the model of whole-person caring, a holistic, spiritually based, interprofessional framework that articulates and operationalizes healing concepts to facilitate individual and organizational transformation. Her work in transforming hospitals into healing environments has received local, state, and national recognition.

She serves on the faculty of Energy Medicine University and is a past president of the American Holistic Nurses Association.

Table of Contents

Preface

One sunny summer morning, a few years ago, I was pushing my grocery cart in a Safeway grocery store in Scottsdale, AZ, when I heard an announcement over the PA system. The hardware store down the street was announcing itself as a "holistic" hardware store. I stopped pushing my cart and said to myself, "Well there you have it. We have done it. Holistic is now a household word." Of course, "they" don't know what holistic means, but it is no longer a bad word.

When we started the American Holistic Medical Association in 1978, it took us another two years to decide how to spell holistic. Spelling it with a W meant something that we were *trying* to say, but spelling it with an H enabled us to share the *real* concept we were hoping to convey. This had to do with the root words associated with holy, healing, and health. In other words, we had to bring the spirit back into the work we were doing. Body, mind, and spirit had to be expressed as one if we were to reclaim the true nature of the healing we knew as our real work.

In some strange way, having the hardware store proclaim itself as "holistic" validated me. I was no longer a "quack," a "witch doctor," a "snake oil salesperson," or something even worse. Rather, I was a holistic doctor. Finally, it could be said publicly—but it took 35 years to get this far. That's okay, though. This is the way life works. You plant a seed and take care of it, and, finally, a little shoot comes up. Now the hard work of cultivating it goes on.

In this book, Lucia Thornton gives us ways by which we can transform the field of health care, which is sick and dying, into a healthy, global garden where healing at all levels can take place and where the caregivers are joyful and healthy and in tune with nature.

When I was in medical school, we were told never to give the patient false hope. When I began working with patients, however, it didn't take long to realize that was wrong. I don't think there is such a thing as false hope. There can be false information and false expectations but not false hope. The Indian poet Tagore said, "Hope is the bird that sings before the dawn." Those of us who work in this field have all seen patients who, against all odds, when given a small ray of hope, improve—and others who were doing well but got worse when that ray of hope was removed.

When qualities of the spirit such as hope, compassion, tenderness, and love are what nurses and other health care providers bring to the field of medicine, healing at all levels becomes a reality. This happens when the patient realizes that the power to heal lies within his or her own being. Our job is to awaken and nurture that healing power within them. We have all watched as a patient who has undergone a beautiful surgery doesn't heal, while another with a botched surgery heals very well. The question is, who does the healing? We need each other.

In my experience, we can deal with many aspects of life, including pain, but we don't deal well with abandonment. No procedure or medication can take the place of another human being. We need each other. As we deal with our own fears, we help others to deal with theirs. We can help others when we know ourselves so that we do not project our fears and pain onto them. None of us are perfect; we are all works in progress. We can share what we have learned.

Just as the hardware store shared with our community its awareness of being holistic, each community shares what it learns. Communities share each others' pain, but they can also share their healing. This book will help us all so that we can become the healing community that helps us to age into health.

–Gladys Taylor McGarey, MD, MD(H)

Foreword

For many years I worked diligently to educate my patients about stress reduction, good nutrition, smoking cessation, and physical fitness. I gradually learned that this approach was, all too frequently, not very successful. Something was missing. Professor Lucia Thornton's brilliant book, *Whole-Person Caring: An Interprofessional Model for Healing and Wellness,* reveals that missing piece. Her book expounds on how the most important ingredient for better health is to better understand and embrace who we are as human beings. I agree with Professor Thornton.

Integrative physicians and nurses have recommended for years that a mind, body, and spirit approach is needed for true healing. Unfortunately, in retrospect, it is easy to see that most of the time healers have neglected the spirit part of that equation. This book gives spirit the significance it deserves, while not avoiding the importance of the body and mind. Thornton understands that there is a divine intelligence in all humans that continually seeks wholeness. When we connect with our higher self, we have a much better chance of finding the inner light that helps us to heal.

One reason I so enjoyed and appreciated this book is because its primary message resonates closely with what routinely occurs by the end of a one-month, fourth-year medical student elective that I teach each year. The elective, which began 12 years ago as a way to develop physician leaders in integrative medicine, teaches students about complementary and alternative medical practices. We soon realized that in addition to learning about such things as nutrition, Chinese and Ayurvedic medicine, and herbs, the students were engaged in a much deeper, more transformative process. These future physicians were experiencing self-reflection, compassion, self-love, the importance of community, and the interconnectedness of all living things.

Year after year, when asked to state the most valuable thing they had learned during the course, these medical students describe how they have primarily learned compassion, how to quiet their minds, and how better to love themselves. They write statements such as, "I learned to be my own person," "I learned to trust my intuition," "I want to dance more," and "I love myself more now."

Thornton, past president of the American Holistic Nurses Association, defines the core problem regarding the U.S. health care system and offers realistic solutions. As stated previously, she believes that we must redefine who we are as human beings, which we do by embracing our energetic and infinite nature. We must reconnect with our spiritual essence. Life is sacred, and the shift to true healing will occur when we see ourselves and each other in that light. Thornton stresses that it is imperative that we bring not just our brains but also our hearts and souls into our lives and our work.

But it is not enough to make just individual changes. A cultural change must also occur in our clinics, hospitals, schools, and lives. Thornton's award-winning whole-person caring model calls forth the highest potential in people and promotes health and healing in individuals and organizations. This multidisciplinary model brings together practitioners from a wide range of healing professions to create a common vision.

Whole-person caring is a powerful reminder that the most important thing we can do to improve health and healing is to remember the spiritual and energetic essence of who we truly are as human beings, to love and trust ourselves, and to remember that we are all connected. There is a divine intelligence in us that continually seeks wholeness. Our job is to remain open to that intelligence and to follow its infinitely wise and loving guidance.

–Bill Manahan, MD
Assistant Professor Emeritus, Department of Family Medicine
University of Minnesota Academic Health Center, Minneapolis, MN
Past President, American Holistic Medical Association
Author of *Eat for Health: Fast and Simple Ways of Eliminating Diseases Without Medical Assistance*

Introduction

"Be the change you wish to see in this world."
—Mahatma Gandhi

How do we reconstruct a health care system that is primarily concerned with disease and illness to include a major focus on health promotion and wellness? How can we integrate healing and caring practices into our hospitals and communities? What are some of the steps that can be taken, and what is the role of nurses and other professionals in this process?

The aim of this book is to present a new way of looking at who we are and what we do. It is about seeing ourselves and our work in a greater light. It is about recognizing our wholeness and recapturing those parts of ourselves that we have left behind. It is about bringing heart and soul back into our lives and work and advocating for a health care system that does the same.

Several years ago, I taught workshops around the United States for nurses interested in holistic nursing. The workshops were transformational in nature. Nurses who attended learned how important it was to care for themselves. They learned that to provide compassionate care and be a healing presence, they must value and care deeply for themselves. The lives of the nurses who attended often changed dramatically. They began to eat more healthfully, get more rest, take breaks at work, exercise, and set aside time for themselves. They began to value who they were, and this made all the difference in the world.

The program involved a mentorship, so I had the opportunity to work and correspond with participants for several months. As I did, I noticed an interesting phenomenon. In the beginning, the nurses were very enthused about their new perspective and excited to bring change and healing to their workplace. They returned to work with wonderful ideas about teamwork, supporting each other, being a healing presence for their patients, and creating a healthy and healing environment. After a month or so, however, their enthusiasm diminished. There simply was no support in their workplaces for such change to occur. Then, two things usually happened: Either they quit nursing because they could no longer tolerate the unhealthy environment, or they reverted to their old ways, settling back into the unhealthy workplace culture.

During this same time period, I worked with several hospitals, offering programs of renewal for their staff. For one hospital, I had the opportunity to offer several "day of renewal" workshops in a row, so that approximately 20% of the medical-surgical staff was able to attend. A month after delivering the program, I received a call from the nurse manager saying that the whole environment in the workplace had changed. She said that doctors who normally came into her office to complain about the nurses were now coming in to compliment the work of her staff. Moreover, she said patient satisfaction had improved dramatically. While I clearly understood the relationship between a healthy and vital workforce and organizational performance, I was skeptical that a 1-day program could create such dramatic changes. I asked the manager if there were other variables that might account for the remarkable shift. Did she hire more staff? Were employees' salaries increased? Was patient acuity down? She replied, "I've been working here for 18 years. I know the staff, and I know the unit. Your day of renewal is the only variable that affected the entire group. *It* has made the difference."

After watching what was happening with the holistic nurses who were disenfranchised shortly after they returned to work, I began to wonder: What if we could get a critical mass of people from a hospital or organization to embrace some of these ideas? Could that create a shift in the culture? When the manager called, I began to think that might have been what happened on the medical-surgical unit.

We observed the patient-satisfaction data, and, after 3 months, the increased levels gradually declined to the previous baseline. Nonetheless, the positive spike caught the attention of the director of clinical services. We began discussing strategies for a sustainable outcome. We realized that to create change in the organizational culture that was sustainable, it was important for the movement to be all-inclusive and all-pervasive. An interdisciplinary approach was imperative. A decision was made to develop a comprehensive program available not only to nurses, but also to other interested staff including respiratory therapists, dieticians, chaplains, administrators, and physicians.

The previous programs were based on nursing theory and designed for nurses. It was necessary to create a model of care to which every discipline could relate and to design an educational program that was interdisciplinary as well. The model of whole-person caring (WPC) was developed and became the foundation for subsequent programs and organizational transformation.

After the model was developed and the in-service programs were offered, nursing turnover significantly decreased and patient satisfaction significantly improved. The hospital saved more than $1.5 million based on the decreased nursing turnover during that year. Additionally, the hospital received local, state, and national recognition for their accomplishments. On a national level, it received the Norman Cousins Award, given by the Fetzer Institute, which acknowledges one health care project each year that significantly focuses on relationships. The hospital received recognition from the state hospital association for excellence in health care leadership and received the regional Innovation in the Workplace Award. The local newspaper also featured many stories related to the healing environment and the compassionate care that the employees provided.

These were all external validations that a caring-healing transformation had taken place. This transformation was something that employees, patients, and the community could actually *feel*. The transformation was led by the nurse manager, the director of clinical services, and a core of staff who understood the concepts of the model of whole-person caring. The model was a guide, but the people did the work. Their story is told in Chapter 4, "Integrating the Model of Whole-Person Caring."

This book is about the model of whole-person caring. The model is an interprofessional and interdisciplinary framework for healing and wellness. It is holistic and spiritual in nature. It is a model that calls forth the highest potential in people and promotes health and healing in people and organizations. It is a model that works.

Several things about the model make it particularly useful in these times. First, it redefines who we are as human beings. It expands the definition of human being beyond the biomedical model to include recent discoveries in science. It acknowledges the infinite and sacred nature of our being. This expanded perspective enables us to look at who we are and what we do in different ways. It invites us to bring healing modalities and therapies into our practices.

Another important aspect of this model is its interdisciplinary and interprofessional orientation. The model was initially developed to serve as an interdisciplinary guide to unite the various disciplines within a hospital in a common framework. These disciplines included professionals (nurses, physicians, dieticians, respiratory therapists, etc.) and other health care employees (nursing assistants, volunteers, clerical staff, maintenance, etc.). The model is equally useful as an interprofessional guide in bringing together people from various health care and healing professions. Professionals from fields such as medicine, nursing, social work, psychology, chiropractics, naturopathy, traditional medical systems, and so on, can utilize the model as a common framework for practice and collaborative care.

This model provides a guide for those who are interested in bringing forth their greatest potential. It sets forth some very high ideals. It is a model that will appeal to people who social science calls *early adopters*. These are the leaders, the visionaries, and those who have already engaged a good portion of their time in personal growth and awakening. For early adopters, this model can help you share with others the vision that you already carry in your heart. It is a model to promote healing and wellness for you, your coworkers, and your organization.

This book also contains practical and useful tools for helping people create healthier and more wholesome ways of being. This book is useful to managers and administrators, but it is equally useful for people wanting to create a healthier lifestyle and bring healing into their lives. The self-care, self-healing, and stress-reducing practices are for everyone, and can serve as a wonderful reference for students, patients, friends, and family. In addition, the descriptions of various complementary and alternative therapies and the various systems of medicine in Chapter 1, "Shifting Toward a Paradigm of Healing and Wellness," can help acquaint those who are not familiar with these practices.

Chapter 1, "Shifting Toward a Paradigm of Healing and Wellness," looks at the current health care system and the need to shift from an illness-based system to a system that is focused on health and wellness. It examines the importance of integrating a holistic approach that values interdisciplinary collaboration and coordination of care. Shifting our resources and our consciousness toward promoting healing and wellness requires people from various service and business sectors to work together. An interdisciplinary framework creates a common vision and provides a common platform from which different disciplines can initiate actions.

Chapter 2, "Redefining Who We Are," examines some of the basic assumptions of the biomedical model. The need to expand our current perspective is asserted. Some of the questions raised in this chapter include: Is the reductionist model that underpins health care practices outdated? Is there a more useful and expansive way of defining ourselves and our universe that creates an openness to healing and interdisciplinary collaboration? How can we see ourselves in a greater light? The chapter discusses recent thinking and research in the field of quantum mechanics, helping to expand our view of who we are. The chapter also examines some of the concepts of nurse theorist Martha Rogers that underpin the definition of person in the model of whole-person caring.

Chapter 3, "The Model of Whole-Person Caring: An Overview," provides a history and basic overview of the definitions and concepts of the model of whole-person caring. The key concepts of whole-person caring—infinite and sacred nature of being; self-compassion, self-care, and self-healing; optimal wellness; therapeutic partnering; transformational leadership; and caring as sacred practice—are discussed. The chapter also explores the importance of an interdisciplinary model that is visionary and sustainable.

Chapter 4, "Integrating the Model of Whole-Person Caring," delineates the process of integrating the model into an organization. Steps include assessing the organization's ideology and culture, eliciting the support of key people, involving everyone, customizing strategies for implementation, honoring and recognizing exemplary people, initiating programs for personal growth and transformation, and incorporating concepts into performance criteria. A manager's case study is presented to show how the model was implemented. The compatibility of the WPC model with other models is also discussed.

Chapter 5, "The Infinite and Sacred Nature of Being," begins the discussion of each of the model's concepts. This chapter focuses on the infinite and sacred nature of being, which is the first concept of the model. It looks at spirituality in health care and at the difference between spirituality and religion. We begin to examine how viewing people as spiritual and infinite beings changes the way we deliver care. What possibilities exist in this framework? What is the potential for healing? We also examine the difference between healing and curing and how the two approaches change the manner in which we provide care. Some steps to integrating spirituality are suggested, including setting the intention, creating the vision, beginning the dialogue, creating reminders, creating healing spaces, developing policies to support a healing environment, and developing and mentoring staff.

Chapter 6, "Self-Compassion, Self-Care, and Self-Healing," discusses the next concepts in the WPC model. Those who are familiar with the model will notice that self-compassion is a new addition. While writing this book, I began to understand the importance of self-compassion as a foundational concept to self-care and self-healing. So the concept of self-compassion has been included along with self-care and self-healing. These concepts are explored, along with practical exercises that you can use to develop compassion toward yourself.

Chapter 7, "Self-Care and Self-Healing Practices," provides the reader with practices and approaches that can be used for self-care and self-healing. You can also share these techniques with family, friends, and coworkers. Some can be used in the clinical setting to help alleviate stress, and can also be taught to patients to help them with pain, sleeplessness, anxiety, and a variety of other problems. You will become acquainted with practices that can alter conscious and unconscious habits, quick and easy ways to de-stress, and breathing exercises to incorporate into your work and personal life. You will also be introduced to some subtle energy practices that will sensitize you to your own energy field and teach you to balance and harmonize the energies in your body.

Chapter 8, "Optimal Health Wellness," explores how to manifest optimal well-being. Optimal wellness involves every aspect of our being. We have been so preoccupied in health care by the disease model that we take little time to imagine how optimal wellness manifests. How does optimal wellness manifest in our mental, emotional, physical, and social/relational life? Because of the rising incidence of obesity and the perpetuation of so many myths about diet and nutrition, special emphasis is given to the area of nutrition. You are provided with basic, up-to-date information to help guide your own nutritional choices and those of your patients. Information is also provided to help you design your own fitness program based on current research.

Chapter 9, "Therapeutic Partnering and Transformational Leadership," explains how to relate to patients and coworkers from a spiritual-energetic base.

Cultivating therapeutic partnerships with our patients helps empower them to take control of their own health. It also creates a field of healing that supports the interaction. Cultivating therapeutic partnerships with our coworkers improves our work relationships and facilitates positive communication and interaction between disciplines in the hospital setting. The importance of developing equitable partnerships as we begin to create integrative models for health care is discussed. The chapter also explores transformational leadership and the healing field of management. The process of cultivating wise leadership is discussed, along with the meaning of spirituality in leadership.

Chapter 10, "Caring as Sacred Practice," examines the last concept of the model, transforming our attitude about caring to include the sacred. How does it change the way we deliver health care when we begin to view all life as sacred? The chapter explains reflective practices that we can use to cultivate our inner healer. Types and techniques of meditation are presented along with a discussion of its importance in cultivating our capacity to heal. Journaling and dream work are also examined. This chapter also teaches techniques that we can incorporate at work to create sacred space and a healing environment. These practices include creating intention, heart centering, and transcendent/transpersonal caring. Some of the research related to these concepts is reviewed, along with the physiological benefits that are associated with these practices.

To borrow from nurse theorist Margaret Newman's terminology, we are at a "choice point" in the way we provide health care. A choice point is preceded by disequilibrium and chaos and creates a realization that our old patterns are ineffective and new ways of doing things must be adopted. While the concept is usually applied to individuals experiencing challenging health issues, this term is quite appropriate for the current state of our health care system. We must find better ways to care for people, promote wellness, and create a sustainable and healthy society.

Nursing is in a unique position to play a major role in the transformation of the health care system. Nurses represent the largest segment of the U.S. health care workforce with more than 3 million members. Nursing practice covers a broad continuum of health care from health promotion, to disease prevention, to coordination of care, to cure when possible, and to palliative care and hospice care when cure is not possible (Institute of Medicine, 2010). This places nurses in a position to play a significant role in the transformation of the health care system.

Nursing alone cannot change the health care paradigm. To create a cultural shift toward health and wellness, the movement must be all-inclusive and all-pervasive. Using an interdisciplinary model that incorporates concepts from nursing, sociology, exercise physiology, stress management, nutrition, psychology, traditional medical systems, and healing practices is a step toward creating a movement that is inclusive.

One of the most important things to remember in this endeavor is this:

> If we are to transform our health care system, we must first transform ourselves.

In the new healing and wellness paradigm, professionals must be role models for healthy and wholesome behaviors. If we are to be advocates for healing and wellness, we ourselves must commit to healthy and wholesome ways of being. This book provides leaders and front-line practitioners in hospitals, schools, and communities with a model to guide their initiatives in creating healthier lives and healthier places to live and work. It is time that we join forces to bring "health" and "care" back into health care! It is time that we become the change we wish to see!

References

Institute of Medicine. (2010). *The future of nursing: Leading change, advancing health.* Robert Woods Johnson Report. Washington, DC: National Academies Press. Retrieved from http://www.nap.edu/openbook.php?record_id=1295

Newman, M. (1994). *Health as expanding consciousness.* Sudberry, MA: Jones and Bartlett.

1

Shifting Toward a Paradigm of Healing and Wellness

"When you're headed in the wrong direction, more speed won't help."

—Anonymous

Where are we headed in health care? The United States is among the wealthiest nations in the world, yet in nearly all indicators of mortality, survival, and life expectancy, it ranks at or near the bottom among high-income countries. Americans live shorter lives and experience more injuries and illnesses than people living in other high-income countries (National Research Council and Institute of Medicine, 2013). If we continue on the same trajectory, almost all trend lines indicate that the U.S. health disadvantages relative to other high-income countries will continue to worsen (ibid., 2013).

Incorporating principles of holism, healing, and wellness into health care practices is necessary to decrease the incidence of chronic disease, to decrease health care costs, and to create a healthier and more vital society. We must alter our direction.

Health Care: An Oxymoron

There are two things missing in our health care system. One is "health", and the other is "care". And herein is the crux of the problem. What does our health care system really do? What does health care really mean? While there are several different definitions of health care, each addresses some aspect of the following (American Heritage Medical Dictionary, 2007; Health care, n.d.; Institute of Medicine, 2010):

- Diagnosis of disease and illness

- Treatment and management of disease and illness

- The restoration and maintenance of health

- The prevention of illness and disease

- The promotion of health and wellness

When people seek health care, it is usually to treat a disease, alleviate symptoms, or care for an acute injury. The places where people typically seek health care are doctors' offices, clinics, and hospitals. People do not seek health care to prevent illness, nor do they regularly seek health care to maintain or manage their health and well-being or for health promotion. Our system primarily addresses diagnosis, treatment, and management of acute and chronic disease and illness. Our system and our practices seldom address the restoration and maintenance of health, the prevention of illness and disease, or the promotion of health. In fact, less than 4% of health care costs are allocated to prevention and public health (Samueli Institute, 2010). Prevention and health promotion do not come to mind when we think of the current health care system.

Returning "Health" to Health Care

Fortunately, there is a movement afoot to put "health" back into health care. There is a growing awareness that our focus must be redirected toward illness prevention and health promotion, largely as a result of the increased incidence of chronic disease. Reports by government and private organizations have emphasized the need to redirect resources for interventions addressing disease prevention and health promotion (Centers for Disease Control and Prevention, 2009; Institute of Medicine, 2001 & 2010; National Research Council and Institute of Medicine, 2013; Samueli Institute, 2010). It is estimated that, as a nation, more than 75% of U.S. health care spending is on people with chronic conditions. The World Health Organization (2013) estimates that if the major risk factors were eliminated, at least 80% of all heart disease, stroke, and type 2 diabetes would be prevented and that more than 40% of cancer would also be prevented.

Initiatives for health promotion, equitable insurance coverage, and illness prevention contained in the 2010 Affordable Care Act have the potential to shift our emphasis away from crisis management and toward wellness. This legislation creates an array of initiatives and funding that provides individuals with improved access to clinical preventative services, provides employers and employees with incentives for workplace wellness initiatives, and creates programs that strengthen the role of communities in promoting prevention. According to Koh and Sebelius (2010, p. 1296), this legislation "will reinvigorate public health on behalf of individuals, worksites, communities, and the nation at large—and will usher in a revitalized era for prevention at every level of society."

Vision for the Future

The committee envisions a future system that makes quality care accessible to the diverse populations of the United States, intentionally promotes wellness and disease prevention, reliably improves health outcomes, and provides compassionate care across the lifespan.

In this envisioned future, primary care and prevention are central drivers of the health care system. Interprofessional collaboration and coordination are the norm. Payment for health care services rewards value, not volume of services, and quality care is provided at a price that is affordable for both individuals and society.

Source: The Institute of Medicine, 2010.

A new vision for health care is emerging. It is a vision that brings health, healing, compassion, and wellness into the conversation. It is a vision that invites professionals to work together to create a healthy and sustainable society. It puts people, their needs, their dreams, and their lives at the core of its efforts. It holds promise and sets us on a course toward a vital and healthy nation.

Integrating Holism in Health Care

A holistic approach can help in our efforts to provide care that fosters optimal health and wellness. Holistic care involves caring for each person as a whole, with an awareness of his or her physical, mental, emotional, and spiritual dimensions and needs.

Holistic care is not a new concept in nursing and medical professions. The precepts of holism are the foundation upon which nursing and medical practices evolved. For example, Florence Nightingale, the founder of modern nursing, was both a scientist and mystic. Hippocrates, the father of Western medicine, was both a physician and priest. These founders understood that the spiritual realms were inseparable from the physical and that all aspects of a person must be considered and brought into harmony for healing to occur.

Holistic care involves a specific body of knowledge and a way of being. It is not just about using various complementary and alternative practices. It values caring, a therapeutic presence, patient empowerment, and healing as foundations when delivering care.

The effectiveness of disease-prevention and health-promotion programs will be determined by how they are implemented, the skills of the providers, and the consciousness and attitudes of the individuals participating in the programs. Programs for prevention and health promotion need to modify people's behavior to be effective. Physical inactivity, poor nutrition, tobacco use, and excessive alcohol consumption are the behaviors responsible for much of the illness, suffering, and early death related to chronic diseases (Centers for Disease Control and Prevention, 2009). However, modifying behavior is not an easy task and necessitates interdisciplinary and holistic strategies using professionals skilled in a variety of approaches. Anyone who has tried to lose weight, commit to an exercise regimen, or change their eating habits understands that there are myriad social and psychological barriers that stand in the way of attaining and maintaining their health goals.

A holistic approach is important to help people modify their behavior. Holistic practitioners are trained to identify behavioral and social patterns contributing to an individual's health challenges, bring these patterns to the individual's awareness, and mutually determine with the person which interventions are appropriate. This is different from the traditional health care model in which the health care practitioner provides patients with a set of instructions or steps to follow without their input and without assessing their readiness to change. Empowering the person to assume control of his or her health is an integral aspect of a holistic approach to care. The relationship between the health care practitioner and the person is a partnership. While the professional offers assessment skills and expertise in interventions, the person decides his or her readiness and chooses which course of action he or she can best pursue.

Holistic practitioners work with people in ongoing relationships that are based in trust and caring. The holistic practitioner follows the person throughout his or her health care challenges and is a therapeutic partner in the person's journey toward health and wellness. Unhealthy behaviors—for instance, those arising from eating and drinking addictions—do not have quick fixes. The underlying motivations for negative behaviors are often longstanding and unconscious. These behaviors will not be changed through the distribution of information about their negative effects. While such information may temporarily shift behaviors, a permanent shift is unlikely to occur unless the underlying cause is dealt with. The holistic practitioner, whether a nurse, physician, social worker, healer, or health coach, understands that a variety of skills and approaches are needed to help a person reach his or her optimal state of health.

The Importance of Interprofessional Collaboration and Coordination of Care

No one professional has all the expertise necessary to help a person with a multitude of social, psychological, and physical problems. Practitioners of conventional medical therapies, mind-body interventions, biologically based therapies, manipulative and body-based methods, exercise and movement programs, and energy therapies can all play a role in helping people achieve optimal health.

The key is coordinating these practitioners to create a system that is focused on health, healing, and wellness. Our health care system has been criticized by consumers, researchers, and numerous commissions over the past decade as ineffective, unaffordable, inaccessible, unorganized, inequitable, and inefficient. The Institute of Medicine reported that the delivery of care is overly complex and uncoordinated, resulting in wasted resources, voids in coverage, loss of information, and a failure to build on the strengths of all health professionals involved to ensure that care is appropriate, timely, and safe (Institute of Medicine, 2001).

Shifting our health care system toward a more holistic model, involving prevention, maintenance, and health promotion, requires input from a broad array of health professionals—physicians, nurses, social workers, psychologists, dieticians, exercise physiologists, physical therapists, and alternative and complementary therapists. Several panels and research committees have emphasized the importance of an interdisciplinary approach in meeting the complex needs of our population. The Institute of Medicine (IOM) reports, "As the delivery of care becomes more complex across a wide range of settings, and the need to coordinate care among multiple providers becomes ever more important, developing well-functioning teams becomes a crucial objective throughout the healthcare system" (2010, p. 72).

Some of the barriers in collaborating among different disciplines include the following:

- Lack of understanding related to what each discipline can contribute

- Mistrust of disciplines outside one's own practice

- Inability to work together in a team approach

- Territorial and reimbursement issues

- Lack of a common model to guide practice

Electronic health records (EHRs) have the potential to help in the coordination of care. Considering the cadre of practitioners involved in a person's care, especially those with chronic illness, a central database allowing easier access to records can eliminate waste (such as the reordering of unnecessary tests and procedures), provide practitioners with complete histories and plans of care, and decrease the ordering of medications that may adversely interact with a person's current prescriptions.

Allowing patients to enter information into their records regarding treatments, programs, and therapies in which they participate outside the conventional health care system will further enhance the process of collaboration. Making certain that people know how to access their own records is important in empowering people to take control of their own health care.

Integrating Healing Practices and Healing Professions into Health Care

There are a wide variety of therapies, modalities, and practices not included in Western medicine that are useful in promoting health and healing. These practices are collectively referred to as *CAM*, which stands for "complementary and alternative medicine." Following are five categories in which these healing therapies can be classified:

- **Botanicals and natural products:** These include natural products such as herbs, vitamins, and mineral supplements, and a variety of herbal and diet therapies.

- **Mind-body-spirit interventions:** Meditation, relaxation, imagery, visualization, hypnosis, yoga, tai chi, prayer, art, music, dance therapies, cognitive-behavioral therapy, biofeedback, therapeutic counseling, aromatherapy, and stress management are included in this category.

- **Manipulative and body-based therapies:** These include chiropractic intervention, massage therapy, osteopathy, reflexology, Alexander technique, and craniosacral therapy.

- **Energy therapies:** Therapeutic touch, Reiki, qigong, acupressure, healing touch, Jyorei, Jin Shin Jyutsu, Pranic healing, light therapy, and magnet therapy are included in this category.

    𝒞ℰ **Whole medical systems:** Traditional Chinese medicine (TCM),
        Ayurveda, osteopathy, homeopathy, naturopathy, and Native Ameri-
        can, Latin American, and African indigenous practices are included.

CAM therapies represent some of the oldest health care interventions used
by people throughout the world. Many of the therapies—whether they are
biologically based, mind-body-spirit practices, physically oriented, or involve
subtle energies—have been used in some form or another by people around
the world since early civilization. The preceding list represents a sampling of
CAM therapies and does not include the entire range of diverse practices. The
descriptions are intended to serve as a brief introduction to acquaint the reader
with some of these practices and therapies.

Botanicals and Natural Products

Botanicals and natural products have been used throughout the world since
the beginning of civilization. Medicinal herbs were found in the personal effects of the mummified "ice man" dating back to prehistoric times. Ancient
Egyptian papyrus writings describe medicinal uses for plants as early as 3000
BCE. Natural products derived from plants, minerals, and animals have been
used by traditional Chinese medicine and Ayurvedic medicine dating back
more than 2,000 years (National Center for Complementary and Alternative
Medicine, 2010b). By the Middle Ages, thousands of botanical products had
been classified for their medicinal effects (National Center for Complementary and Alternative Medicine, 2011).

The World Health Organization (2008) reports that herbal treatments are the
most popular form of traditional medicine. In Germany, between 600 and 700
plant-based medicines are produced and prescribed by 70% of German physicians. In the past 2 decades in the United States, public frustration with the
expense of prescription medications, combined with an interest in returning

to natural or organic remedies, has increased the use of herbs and supplements (Ehrlich, 2011b). The number of adults in the United States who had ever used herbs or supplements grew from 50.6 million in 2002 to 55.1 million in 2007 (Wu, Wang, & Kennedy, 2011).

The most commonly used herbal supplements in the United States include Echinacea, St. John's wort, ginkgo, garlic, saw palmetto, ginseng, goldenseal, valerian, chamomile, feverfew, ginger, evening primrose, and milk thistle. Herbal medicine is used to treat many conditions, including asthma, eczema, premenstrual syndrome, rheumatoid arthritis, migraine, menopausal symptoms, chronic fatigue, irritable bowel syndrome, and cancer. In addition, approximately one fourth of prescription drugs come from plants (Ehrlich, 2011b).

Mind-Body-Spirit Interventions

The oldest forms of mind-body-spirit interventions are the use of prayer, meditation, and yoga, whose origins date back 5,000 years in ancient India. Prior to the 1700s, virtually every medical system in the world treated the mind, body, and spirit as a whole. People were believed to be participants in an interconnected universe (University of Minnesota, 2013).

The science of psychoneuroimmunology (PNI) studies the interaction between behavior, emotional states, the nervous system, the endocrine system, and the immune system (Ehrlich, 2012). Research in this field validates the unity of the body and the mind, showing that all the cells of our body are affected by our thoughts and our beliefs (Pert, 1999; Lipton, 2005). For example, research has shown that stress related to hostility and anxiety can result in disruptions in heart and immune function. Likewise, depression and distress can decrease the body's natural capacity to heal (Ehrlich, 2012).

The usage of mind-body-spirit therapies is now widespread. Mind-body-spirit programs have been established at many medical schools in the United States and around the world. Holistic nurses regularly employ imagery, visualization, relaxation, deep-breathing techniques, stress management, and prayer in caring for patients in hospitals and private practice.

Mind-body-spirit techniques are useful to many conditions because they encourage relaxation, improve coping skills, reduce tension and pain, and lessen the need for medication. Symptoms of anxiety and depression also respond well to mind-body-spirit techniques (Ehrlich, 2012).

Manipulative and Body-Based Therapies

The use of manipulative and body-based therapies dates back to early civilizations. Tui na massage, considered the oldest form of massage, dates back 4,000 years in Chinese medical literature and continues to be an important component of TCM. Tui na massage uses different massage and manipulative techniques along with moxibustion and cupping. It is a major component of TCM and is one of the primary therapies offered in TCM hospitals throughout China (Thornton, 2012). Reflexology, a form of foot and hand massage, is believed to have been practiced more than 4,000 years ago in ancient Egypt, as evidenced by illustrations found on the wall at Saqqara, Egypt, dating to around 2330 BCE (Universal College of Reflexology, n.d.).

Massage is one of the most widely used therapies in the United States. It is rather amusing that massage is listed among alternative and complementary therapies, especially when one considers that just 30 years ago it was considered a part of the routine evening care that nurses provided for patients. Research supports the notion that massage therapy is effective for reducing anxiety, depression, and musculoskeletal pain, and for decreasing blood pressure and heart rate (National Center for Complementary and Alternative Medicine, 2010a).

A plethora of different body and movement therapies has been developed over the last century. Rolfing, developed by Ida Pauline Rolfing in the 1930s, is a form of deep-tissue massage. In the early 1900s, F. M. Alexander developed a technique to guide people to improve their posture and movement and to use their muscles more efficiently (The Complete Guide to the Alexander Technique, n.d.). Moshe Feldenkrais, MD, developed a method to improve the coordination of the whole person in comfortable, effective, and intelligent movement (Wildman & Stephens, 2007). All of these therapies have much anecdotal research confirming their positive effects in reducing anxiety, alleviating stress, and helping and/or correcting musculoskeletal problems.

Energy Therapies

Energy therapies can be grouped into two categories:

- **Veritable:** These involve fields of energy that can be measured.

- **Putative or subtle:** These involve fields of energy that cannot be measured.

The measurable, or veritable, practices include the use of electromagnetic fields such as magnetic and light therapy. The subtle energy therapies include practices such as acupuncture, healing touch, therapeutic touch, Reiki, qigong, and Pranic healing (National Center for Complementary and Alternative Medicine, 2011).

Acupuncture, one of the most widely used and researched practices, has been integrated into many hospitals and clinics. Acupuncture is particularly effective for pain relief and for nausea and vomiting after surgery or chemotherapy. Both the World Health Organization and the National Institutes of Health recognize that acupuncture can be a helpful part of a treatment plan for many illnesses including addiction, asthma, bronchitis, carpal tunnel syndrome, constipation, diarrhea, facial tics, fibromyalgia, headaches, irregular menstrual cycles, polycystic ovarian syndrome, low back pain, menopausal symptoms, menstrual cramps, osteoarthritis, sinusitis, spastic colon (often called *irritable bowel syndrome*), stroke rehabilitation, tendinitis, tennis elbow, and urinary problems such as incontinence (Ehrlich, 2011a).

There are hundreds of different forms of subtle energy therapies that are practiced throughout the world. These practices are based on the assumption that human beings are complex fields of energy. Each practice is shaped by the beliefs and experiences of the founders, and many methods are modified as practitioners develop their own style. In the last several decades, there has been a greater proliferation of subtle energy therapies than ever before. Some of these practices have been passed down through many generations of healers; others were developed within the last 30 years. Some of the more common forms that are practiced in the United States include therapeutic touch, healing touch, Reiki, qigong, Jin Shin Jyutsu, Jyorei, Pranic healing, and polarity therapy. Of these, healing touch, therapeutic touch, and Reiki are the forms that are most commonly practiced by nurses. Healing touch and therapeutic touch were developed by nurses and offer certification and credentialing. The standardization of training and skills obtained through the healing touch and therapeutic touch programs makes their integration into hospitals more accepted than other forms of healing that are passed down through oral tradition.

There have been numerous studies related to the effects of subtle energy therapies. These therapies have been shown to be useful in reducing stress, pain, and anxiety; accelerating healing; and promoting a greater sense of well-being (Wardell, 2004; Monroe, 2009; Zolfagharis, Eypoosh, & Hazrati, 2012). People experiencing energy therapies for the first time often comment on how relaxed and peaceful they feel.

There has been difficulty, however, in designing research that meets the mindset of modern science. Subtle energies, consciousness, and healing are not phenomena that lend themselves well to randomly controlled double-blind studies. New ways of designing research and an openness to new paradigms are important to advance the integration of healing practices. Perhaps it is time to shift from a mantra of "evidence-based practice" to one of "practice-based evidence" (D. W. Wardell, personal communication, November 6, 2004). We have advocated in recent years for patient-centered care; it may be time to advocate for patient-centered research.

Whole Medical Systems

Whole medical systems are complete systems of theory and practice that have developed independently from or parallel to Western medicine. Many alternative medical systems have been practiced by individual cultures throughout the world. Major Eastern whole medical systems include TCM and Ayurveda and date back more than 5,000 years. Major Western whole medical systems that have developed in the last century include homeopathy, naturopathy, and osteopathy. Other whole medical systems have been developed by Native American, Tibetan, and Central- and South-American cultures. The following is a sampling of Eastern and Western whole medical systems.

Traditional Chinese Medicine

TCM, rooted in the ancient philosophy of Taoism, has a rich and long history dating back more than 5,000 years. TCM remained isolated from the world until China opened up in 1972. Gradually, TCM spread to the United States and Western medicine spread to China.

In China, there are hospitals that primarily practice Western medicine and hospitals that mostly practice TCM. There is some integration of the two systems in each of the hospitals. For instance, if a person were admitted to a Western-medicine hospital with a bone fracture, the bone would be set and cast; then, an acupuncturist on staff would visit the person in the hospital and give several treatments to stimulate bone repair and healing. Likewise, if a person were admitted to a TCM hospital with acute pain of unknown origin, the TCM hospital might use a CT scan or MRI for diagnosis and then proceed to treat according to TCM principles (Thornton, 2012).

TCM is used widely in the United States. It was estimated in 1997 that some 10,000 practitioners served more than 1 million patients each year. According to the 2007 National Health Interview Survey, an estimated 3.1 million U.S. adults reported using acupuncture in the previous year. In another survey, more than one third of the patients at six large acupuncture clinics said they also received Chinese herbal treatments at the clinics (National Center for Complementary and Alternative Medicine, 2010b).

The cornerstone of TCM is its effectiveness in keeping people healthy. Maintaining a balance between *yin* and *yang* is a foundational concept in TCM. *Yin* and *yang* are considered opposites. The TCM practitioner works with people to bring these energies into balance through diet modification, herbs, acupuncture, massage, and energy practices such as qigong or tai chi. TCM diagnosis uses inspection of tongue, complexion, posture, auscultation, pulse taking, and history (Nan, 2012).

Ayurvedic Medicine

Ayurvedic medicine, one of the oldest medical systems in the world, provides a holistic approach to health that is designed to help people live long, healthy, and well-balanced lives. The goal of Ayurvedic medicine is to prevent diseases (Ehrlich, 2011a).

Ayurvedic medicine has several key principles that pertain to health and disease. These concepts relate to universal interconnectedness, the body's constitution (*prakriti*), and life forces (*doshas*). Ayurvedic treatment is individualized to each person's constitution. Practitioners expect patients to be active participants because many Ayurvedic treatments require changes in diet, life-style, and habits. Ayurvedic treatment goals include eliminating impurities, reducing symptoms, increasing resistance to disease, reducing worry, and increasing harmony in people's lives (National Center for Complementary and Alternative Medicine, 2009).

The United States has no national standard for training or certifying Ayurvedic practitioners, although a few states have approved Ayurvedic schools as educational institutions. According to the 2007 National Health Interview Survey, which included a comprehensive survey of CAM use by Americans, more than 200,000 U.S. adults had used Ayurvedic medicine in the previous year (National Center for Complementary and Alternative Medicine, 2009).

Naturopathy

Naturopathy is a system of medicine based on the healing power of nature. The aim of naturopathy is to support the body's ability to heal itself through the use of dietary and lifestyle changes, herbal medicine, and detoxification. Naturopathic doctors (NDs) treat the whole person, assessing the person's mental, emotional, and spiritual state; diet; family history; environment; and lifestyle before making a diagnosis.

Naturopaths treat both acute and chronic conditions, from arthritis to ear infections, from HIV to asthma, from congestive heart failure to hepatitis. NDs treat the whole person rather than treating a disease or its symptoms only, aiming to help their patients maintain a balanced state of good health. Because of this holistic approach, naturopathy is especially suited for treating chronic illnesses (Ehrlich, 2011d).

Osteopathy

Osteopathy, based on the belief that most diseases are related to problems in the musculoskeletal system, was founded in 1874 by Andrew Taylor Still. The American Osteopathic Association was formed in 1902; in 1962, doctors of osteopathy (DOs) were given full practice rights in all 50 states. In addition to acquiring the same basic training as MDs, DOs are taught how to perform manipulative adjustments (Ehrlich, 2011e). Osteopaths believe that the body possesses self-regulatory and self-healing mechanisms and that the body is a single dynamic unit of function (The Osteopathic Academy, n.d.).

Homeopathy

Homeopathy is a holistic system of treatment established in 1796 by the German physician Samuel Christian Hahnemann. It treats people with heavily diluted preparations of substances, which, in their undiluted form, are thought to cause effects similar to the symptoms presented—a phenomenon called the *Law of Similars* (World Health Organization, 2009). Homeopathic remedies are believed to stimulate the body's own healing processes.

The purpose of homeopathy is to restore the body to a healthy balance. The symptoms of a disease are regarded as the body's own defensive attempt to correct its imbalance. A homeopath regards symptoms as evidence of the body's inner intelligence and prescribes a remedy to stimulate this internal curative process rather than suppress the symptoms. In homeopathy, the curative process extends beyond the relief of immediate symptoms of illness. Healing may come in many stages, as the practitioner treats layers of symptoms believed to be remnants of traumas or chronic disease in the person's past (Homeopathic medicine, n.d.).

An initial visit to a homeopathic physician will take one to two hours. The homeopath performs a *case-taking* to get a complete picture of a person's general health and lifestyle, as well as particular symptoms on the physical, mental, and emotional levels. Homeopathic practitioners believe that illness is specific to an individual. For instance, two people with the same symptoms will often receive different remedies based on their constitution. A person's constitution includes qualities related to creativity, initiative, persistence, concentration, physical sensitivities, and stamina (Homeopathic medicine, n.d.; Ehrlich, 2011c).

Preliminary evidence shows that homeopathy may be helpful in treating childhood diarrhea, otitis media, asthma, fibromyalgia, chronic fatigue syndrome, symptoms of menopause (such as hot flashes), pain, allergies, upper respiratory tract infections, sore muscles, and colds and flu (Ehrlich, 2011c).

Summary

Health care in the United States has focused on treatment of disease and illness, with little emphasis on health promotion and disease prevention. National awareness and efforts to redirect health care toward illness prevention and health promotion have accelerated due to the increased incidence and high cost of chronic disease, which is largely preventable.

A holistic approach that considers all aspects of a person is important in changing behaviors and creating healthy lifestyles. Empowering people to take control of their lives and creating ongoing relationships based in trust and caring are essential. An interdisciplinary approach that is well coordinated is necessary to provide support in meeting the diverse needs of the chronically ill and for health promotion.

Integrating healing therapies into health care practices is useful and often provides cost-effective alternatives to Western medicine. Referred to as *complementary and alternative medicine (CAM)*, these therapies represent some of the oldest health care interventions used by people throughout the world.

Mind-body-spirit therapies such as prayer, meditation, yoga, affirmations, imagery, and visualization have been useful in a variety of conditions because of their capability to encourage relaxation, improve coping skills, and reduce tension and pain. Massage and other body therapies are useful in reducing anxiety, depression, and musculoskeletal pain. Likewise, subtle energy therapies have been shown to be useful in reducing stress, pain, and anxiety; accelerating healing; and promoting a greater sense of well-being.

Medical systems—such as traditional Chinese medicine, Ayurvedic medicine, naturopathy, homeopathy, and osteopathy—that treat the whole person have valuable contributions to make to our health care system. They focus on prevention, patient empowerment, healthy lifestyles, and the rare utilization of high-cost interventions. This places these systems in a position to help shift health care toward a paradigm of health, healing, and wellness, and provide affordable and sustainable care.

A new vision for health care is emerging. It is a vision that brings health, healing, compassion, and wellness into the conversation. It is a vision that invites professionals to work together to create a healthy and sustainable society. It puts people, their needs, their dreams, and their lives at the core of its efforts. It holds promise and sets us on a course toward a vital and healthy society.

References

American Heritage Medical Dictionary. (2007). Accessed on January 30, 2013 from http://medical-dictionary.thefreedictionary.com/health+care

Centers for Disease Control and Prevention. (2009). The power of prevention: Chronic disease…the public health challenge of the 21st century. Retrieved from http://www.cdc.gov/chronicdisease/pdf/2009-Power-of-Prevention.pdf

The Complete Guide to the Alexander Technique. (n.d.). Who was Frederick Matthias Alexander? Retrieved from http://www.alexandertechnique.com/fma.htm

Ehrlich, S. D. (2011a). Acupuncture. *University of Maryland Medical Center*. Retrieved from http://www.umm.edu/altmed/articles/acupuncture-000345.htm#ixzz2J1mkuTkn

Ehrlich, S. D. (2011b). Herbal medicine. *University of Maryland Medical Center*. Retrieved from http://www.umm.edu/altmed/articles/herbal-medicine-000351.htm#ixzz2IYHElEgL

Ehrlich, S. D. (2011c). Homeopathy. *University of Maryland Medical Center.* Retrieved from http://www.umm.edu/altmed/articles/homeopathy-000352.htm

Ehrlich, S. D. (2011d). Naturopathy. *University of Maryland Medical Center.* Retrieved from http://www.umm.edu/altmed/articles/naturopathy-000356.htm

Ehrlich, S. D. (2011e). Osteopathy. *University of Maryland Medical Center.* Retrieved from http://www.umm.edu/altmed/articles/osteopathy-000358.htm

Ehrlich, S. D. (2012). Mind-body medicine. *University of Maryland Medical Center.* Retrieved from http://www.umm.edu/altmed/articles/mind-body-000355.htm

Health care. (n.d.). In *Merriam-Webster's online dictionary* (11th ed.). Retrieved from http://www.merriam-webster.com/dictionary/healthcare

Homeopathic medicine. (n.d.) In *The Free Dictionary by Farlex.* Retrieved from http://medical-dictionary.thefreedictionary.com/Homeopathic+Medicine

Institute of Medicine. (2001). Crossing the quality chasm: A new health system for the 21st century. Retrieved from http://iom.edu/~/media/Files/Report%20Files/2001/Crossing-the-Quality-Chasm/Quality%20Chasm%202001%20%20report%20brief.pdf

Institute of Medicine. (2010). *The future of nursing: Leading change, advancing health.* Robert Woods Johnson Report. Washington, DC: National Academies Press. Retrieved from http://www.nap.edu/openbook.php?record_id=1295

Koh, H. K., & Sebelius, K. (2010). Promoting prevention through the affordable care act. *The New England Journal of Medicine, 363*(14), 1296–1299. doi: 10.1056/NEJMp1008560

Lipton, B. (2005). *The biology of belief: Unleashing the power of consciousness, matter and miracles.* Santa Rosa, CA: Elite Books.

Monroe, C. M. (2009). The effects of therapeutic touch on pain. *Journal of Holistic Nursing, 27*(2), 85–92.

Nan, J. (2012, October). Presentation to healing traditions delegation. *People to people ambassador program.* Symposium conducted at the Guang'anmen Traditional Chinese Medicine Hospital, Beijing, China.

National Center for Complementary and Alternative Medicine. (2009). Ayurvedic medicine: An introduction. Retrieved from http://nccam.nih.gov/health/ayurveda/introduction.htm

National Center for Complementary and Alternative Medicine. (2010a). Massage therapy: An introduction. Retrieved from http://nccam.nih.gov/health/massage/massageintroduction.htm

National Center for Complementary and Alternative Medicine. (2010b). Traditional Chinese medicine: An introduction. Retrieved from http://nccam.nih.gov/health/whatiscam/chinesemed.htm

National Center for Complementary and Alternative Medicine. (2011). What is complementary and alternative medicine? Retrieved from http://nccam.nih.gov/health/whatiscam

National Research Council and Institute of Medicine. (2013). *U.S. health in international perspective: Shorter lives, poorer health.* Washington, DC: The National Academies Press. http://www.nap.edu/catalog.php?record_id=134

The Osteopathic Academy. (n.d.). Philosophical foundations of osteopathy. Retrieved from http://www.cranialacademy.com/philosophy.html

Pert, C. (1999). *Molecules of emotion.* New York, NY: Simon & Schuster.

Samueli Institute (2010). *A wellness initiative for the nation.* Retrieved from http://www.samueliinstitute.org/health-policy/wellness-initiative-for-the-nation-win

Thornton, L. (2012). The healing traditions delegation to China. *People to People Ambassador Program Journal of Professional Proceeding*s. Retrieved from http://citizens.peopletopeople.com/PTP%20Documents/Citizen%20Programs/Journals/Medicine/Thornton_Journal_7540_7749.pdf

Universal College of Reflexology. (n.d.). History of foot and hand reflexology. http://www.universalreflex.com/article.php/20040315123726347

University of Minnesota. (2010). Mind-body therapies [Web log post]. Retrieved from http://takingcharge.csh.umn.edu/explore-healing-practices/what-are-mind-body-therapies

Wardell, D W. (2004). Review of studies of healing touch. *Journal of Nursing Scholarship, 36*(2), 147–154.

Wildman, F., & Stephens, J. (2007). Origins and history. *Feldenkrais Movement Institute.* Retrieved from http://www.feldenkraisinstitute.org/articles/a_origins.html

World Health Organization. (2008). Traditional medicine. Retrieved from http://www.who.int/mediacentre/factsheets/fs134/en/

World Health Organization. (2009). Safety issues in the preparation of homeopathic medicines. Retrieved from www.who.int/entity/medicines/areas/traditional/Homeopathy.pdf

World Health Organization. (2013). Chronic diseases and health promotion. Retrieved from http://www.who.int/chp/chronic_disease_report/part1/en/index11.html

Wu, C. H., Wang, C. C., & Kennedy, J. (2011). Changes in herb and dietary supplement use in the U.S. adult population: A comparison of the 2002 and 2007 national health interview surveys. *Journal of Clinical Therapies,* (11), 1749–58. doi: 10.1016/j.clinthera.2011.09.024

Zolfagharis, M., Eypoosh, S., & Hazrati, M. (2012). Effects of therapeutic touch on anxiety, vital signs, and cardiac dysrhythmia in a sample of Iranian women undergoing cardiac catheterization. *Journal of Holistic Nursing, 30*(4), 225–234.

2

Redefining Who
We Are

*"We are all elements of spirit, indestructible
and eternal, and multiplexed in the divine."*

*–William A. Tiller, PhD, Professor
Emeritus Stanford University*

Defining who we are is the first step in establishing a
model of care. The way we perceive ourselves as human beings guides our practice, our research, and ultimately our
body of knowledge. The way we define ourselves is one of
the deepest underlying assumptions in a culture. Assumptions at this level are often taken for granted and are not
usually articulated. However, deeply rooted assumptions are
what affect why things happen or fail to happen in a culture
(Carroll & Quijada, 2004).

Current Biomedical View

The biomedical model that guides health care practices today has its origin in the mechanistic and reductionist thinking of the 17th century. In this model, guided by the discoveries and theories of such notables as Descartes and Newton, people are perceived to be the amalgamation of molecules and atoms that interact in a predictable fashion based on laws of mathematics, chemistry, and physics (Curtis & Gaylord, 2004). What can be seen, dissected, examined, and quantified are the phenomena of interest in modern medicine. This approach is responsible for many of the wondrous advances in medicine and health care over the last century. The advents of antibiotics, vaccinations, anesthesia, DNA research, advanced imaging, surgical interventions, and organ transplants, to name a few, are the products of mechanistic and reductionist methodology. It is a way of thinking, practicing, and perceiving that is deeply embedded in the health care and scientific communities.

The problem is that deeply held assumptions are not questioned, and they become less and less open to discussion over time (Schein, 1990). In his classic book *The Structure of Scientific Revolutions* (1996), Thomas Kuhn asserted that the dominant scientific paradigm will govern the thinking of entire generations of scientists and teach them what is worth investigating and what is not.

Once a paradigm is embedded, it creates filters that determine what a scientific community sees and, consequently, what research will be pursued and what results will be lauded and published. So it is with the predominant biomedical view of human beings in our culture. Considering that the reductionist perspective has been prominent for the past three centuries, it is little wonder that any ideas outside the norm can gain acceptance. Realizing the long history and deeply embedded nature of this perception helps explain the resistance to concepts that threaten to change or expand the definition of who we are. While this perspective has been extremely useful, it falls short in explaining many of the phenomena and practices associated with healing. It does not fully describe who we are, and it needs to be expanded if we are to evolve toward a healing paradigm.

The Need to Expand Our Perspective

There are several reasons why it is useful to expand our notion of who we are. First, the idea that we are simply biomedical entities does not meet the criteria needed for a valid scientific concept. Listed here are five elements that most people want a scientific body of knowledge to provide (Reynolds, 1971):

- A method of organizing and categorizing "things" (a typology)
- Predictions of future events
- Explanations of past events
- A sense of understanding about what causes events
- The potential for control of events

How does the biomedical model measure up to meeting these criteria? Let's look at acupuncture in relation to these objectives. There is a large body of research that substantiates the effectiveness of acupuncture in alleviating pain. If one views a person as a composite of separate neurons, cells, organs, systems, and senses, there is no explanation of how or why acupuncture could or should work. Receiving pain relief by placing needles in various parts of the body that are not connected to the area that is symptomatic is incongruent with the current medical paradigm. Within the biomedical model, acupuncture makes no sense. Yet, it works!

In this case, a reductionist perspective fails to meet the three criteria of predicting, explaining, and giving us a sense of understanding about the intervention. The same could be applied to interventions involving subtle energy therapies, homeopathy, aromatherapy, reflexology, traditional Chinese medicine, Ayurvedic medicine, and an array of other practices and systems of medicine. Too many phenomena occur that cannot be predicted, explained, or understood within the context of the biomedical model. Thus, a primary reason that we need to expand our perspective beyond the mechanistic reductionist view is to meet the criteria for a valid scientific concept. It's simply good science. Bad science, on the other hand, is looking at all these interventions and saying, "Because they are not predictable, are not explainable, or cannot be understood by the current paradigm, they are not worth considering or using." It is not the interventions that are flawed; it is the paradigm!

Expanding our perspective makes way for a larger body of knowledge and healing practices to be accepted into our health care system. Research has proved the effectiveness of many traditional healing practices and therapies in alleviating or ameliorating a variety of symptoms and illnesses. When healing practices—especially those involving subtle energies—are viewed through the lens of reductionist sciences, there is often no "mechanism of action" that can be deciphered. Consequently, the predicted response from anyone educated and practicing in the biomedical system is to ignore, dismiss, and/or ridicule the interventions as fraudulent. The biomedical practitioner cannot entertain the idea that these practices might have a therapeutic effect; it is literally out of his or her paradigm. Also, research into these practices is sometimes ignored or dismissed as invalid either because the research design does not conform to the rigors of a randomized controlled study or because the results of the data make no sense within the reductionist world view. Expanding our current perspective to one that can explain phenomena beyond the biomedical view will help in the acceptance and advancement of many efficacious healing practices.

Further, a reductionist perspective is inadequate for dealing with the increasing prevalence of chronic disease and the promotion of wellness. A person with chronic disease or diseases has a multitude of interrelated factors that affect his or her condition. The current biomedical system views who we are as an amalgamation of parts cared for by a variety of specialists. A holistic perspective that takes into consideration the inseparability and interrelatedness of the mental, emotional, physical, and social-relational aspects of a person is crucial in delivering effective care for the complex issues facing the chronically ill. A holistic approach that integrates practices that foster health and wholeness is crucial in shifting our health care system from a disease and illness orientation toward one of health promotion and wellness.

Experiences as a Young Nurse

As a young nurse, I cared for two patients who forever changed the limited way that I perceived who we are as human beings and opened my mind to alternative paradigms and world views.

The first patient was a middle-aged man, Mr. Smith, who was admitted to the hospital for an appendectomy. I was a student nurse and had been assigned to care for Mr. Smith for several days. Mr. Smith recovered well from his surgery, but the day before he was to be discharged, he said to me, "I think that we should say our good-byes before you leave today." I replied, "Mr. Smith, that won't be necessary! I'll be here tomorrow to discharge you." He was very persistent and acknowledged that even though I would be there early in the morning, it would be best to say our good-byes before I left that day. While I felt it was quite premature, we said our good-byes. When I said "I'll see you tomorrow," he didn't reply, but gently nodded his head and smiled.

When I returned to the hospital the next day, I was informed in report that Mr. Smith had died. How could that be? His vital signs were stable. His blood work was normal. The surgical incision was healing well. He had no history of cardiac problems. There was no evidence of any blood clotting or respiratory distress. When I left Mr. Smith, he was perfectly fine—except that somehow, he knew he was going to die! How did he know? Where did that knowingness come from? If we are just biomedical entities, how can we possibly have the capacity for this type of premonition—especially when it contradicts quantifiable data? Mr. Smith helped me understand that there was much more to who we are than meets the observable eye.

The second patient who changed my perception was Mr. Cohen. Mr. Cohen was in his late sixties and had suffered a massive stroke. He was admitted to the intensive care unit, was placed on a respirator, and had been unconscious and unresponsive to any stimuli for several days. His neurologist had performed two electroencephalograms (EEGs) to determine the extent of brain damage. Both of the EEGs showed that Mr. Cohen had no brainwave activity.

I was working the night shift. It was the eve of Yom Kippur. The neurologist and internist were at Mr. Cohen's bedside, discussing the latest EEG results. They agreed that there was no hope for Mr. Cohen because both EEGs confirmed that there was no brain activity. Mr. Cohen's family was brought in, and the decision was made to wait until after Yom Kippur to take him off the respirator. Being Jewish, the family did not want Mr. Cohen to die on Yom Kippur, the Day of Atonement. As I was listening to this conversation and watching Mr. Cohen, I had a sense that, in spite of his flat EEGs, he was somehow conscious of what was happening.

After the family and his physicians left, I stood by Mr. Cohen's bedside, held his hand, and said, "It must be awfully frightening to hear people talking about taking you off the respirator and about dying." As I stood there holding his hand, I looked at his face and saw a tear falling down Mr. Cohen's cheek. Mr. Cohen was there! That night, I spent every spare moment at Mr. Cohen's bedside, talking to him, massaging his arms, holding his hand, and just being with him as much as possible. When the morning shift arrived for report, Mr. Cohen opened his eyes! He was extubated the following day and sent to a medical surgical floor, where he remained for two weeks before being discharged.

How was this possible? How did someone regain consciousness after he had been diagnosed as brain dead? What *is* consciousness? Can our consciousness exist outside and separate from our brain and body? Fully recovering when there has been no evidence of any brain activity simply does not make sense if we view ourselves as biomedical entities. Mr. Cohen helped me understand that we are more that an amalgamation of biological, physiological, and psychological functions. He taught me that our consciousness can exist outside the function of our brains—that there is something much greater that defines who we are, and there is certainly something more that enlivens us.

Our past experiences shape the way we view the world. These are examples of experiences that challenged my view of who we are and allowed me to entertain other possibilities. Without experiences like these, it might be very difficult to entertain the possibility that other perspectives are valid.

Changing Paradigms

Changing paradigms—especially when it causes us to change the way we view who we are and how the world around us functions—does not come easily. Change is resisted by most and welcomed by few. Thus, to propose a major paradigm shift as the solution to our current health care dilemma is not an idea that will be readily accepted. And yet, a major paradigmatic shift is necessary if we are to integrate practices and ways of being that foster health and wholeness in our health care system and in our society.

I once heard a theologian say that there are three perceptions of who we are: how we perceive ourselves, how others perceive us, and who we really are. One of the greatest challenges in life, he said, is to bring these three perceptions together. What does this mean for us living in our current paradigm?

Our current biomedical paradigm basically sees the physical body as the only dimension of human existence. This is what has been valued, believed, and consecrated for the past 300 years. Scientific technology has driven the innovations and discoveries for the last three centuries. And mechanistic science has been the gatekeeper for the repository of knowledge upon which medicine and health care is based. So, essentially, the collective mind of society has been embedded with the perception that *who we are is our body*. Moreover, 99% of all that is contained in our official body of knowledge is based on this premise.

This idea that *we are only our bodies* is one of the deepest underlying assumptions in our scientific culture. As was stated earlier, assumptions at this level are what affect why things happen or fail to happen in a culture. It may seem like a silly philosophical pursuit to redefine who we are, but unless we do, we cannot move forward in our thinking.

We Cannot Measure What Enlivens Us

The most profound and remarkable experiences in our lives can never be captured in a double-blind study. Love, the *aha* moments of realization felt when standing on top of a mountain—these are not things that can be predicted. Moments that have brought us great joy, moments that have brought us to our knees, moments of mystical experience and spiritual awakening—these are not experiences that can be reduced and analyzed. They are not things that can be explained or predicted. Yet they are the very things that enliven us—the things that give meaning to our lives, and the things that make us happy and whole.

Our current science cannot measure what is important in life. It cannot capture love. It cannot capture healing. So our science says, "If we cannot measure it, it is not real." But anyone who has ever loved or been healed will never be convinced that their experience was not real. The mechanistic/materialistic model that has guided our practice, our lives, and our evolution for the past

300 years has little room in its conceptual framework for ideas like love, joy, hope, compassion, and healing. These things don't fit. They are difficult to measure. They can't be reduced, nor can they be predicted.

The very things that make us happy and healthy are the things that are rejected by the prevailing scientific paradigm. And this is where we must start if we are to begin to create a better world. Our thinking and our consciousness must expand to embrace that which we have rejected. The separation of body, mind, heart, and spirit that occurred in our thinking several hundred years ago was useful in many respects. Just as children separate from their parents to form their own egoic and personality structure in order to function in the world, so, too, the emphasis on the body and all things material has allowed society to advance technologically and materialistically. We are at a point, however, where unless we begin to acknowledge and value our heart and spirit, we will be like the child who has incredible capabilities yet cannot interact and function in the world. We must recover our heart and spirit.

Moving Toward an Einsteinian Perspective

As physicists have recognized, the reality of who we are is too rich to be fully expressed in any model or theory (Harmon, 1998). In our quest to find out who we really are, we must approach this pursuit knowing that we shall fall short. We will never be able to define or capture the complete essence of self. The intention is to shift our perception so that our definition can begin to capture some of the aspects of ourselves that have been left out.

Einstein reportedly said, "Whether you can observe a thing or not depends on the theory which you use. It is the theory which decides what can be observed" (Salam, 1990). The intention of our definition is to expand our perspective so that those things in life that make us happy, healthy, and whole can be observed and acknowledged. Creating a definition that has the capacity to explain the phenomena associated with subtle energies and healing is not only useful, but also necessary to create a paradigm of health, healing, and wellness.

In his classic book *Vibrational Medicine*, Richard Gerber talks about moving from a Newtonian model of medicine to an Einsteinian view. Einstein, through his famous equation $E=mc^2$, postulated that energy and matter are dual expressions of the same universal substance. Mass and energy, although different, are both manifestations of the same thing. We are all composed of this universal substance, this primal energy. While the Einsteinian view has slowly found acceptance and application in the minds of physicists, Einstein's profound insights have yet to be incorporated into the way physicians look at human beings (Gerber, 2001).

We all learned in basic science that all matter is composed of atoms. What we may not have learned or remembered is that atoms are composed of more than 99.9999% empty space, and the center of an atom, the nucleus, is only a trillionth of a centimeter across. The rest of the atom is entirely empty space with a few neutrons, photons, quarks, leptons, gluons, and their corresponding antiparticles dancing about in a subatomic dance (Lawrence Berkeley National Laboratory, 2012). If you removed all the empty space from the atoms that make up all the humans on the planet, you could fit all 6 billion people inside a single apple (Sen, 2007). Even in an altered state of consciousness, that is hard to fathom!

So what fills all this empty space inside of us and the rest of the universe? Craig Hogan, the director of the Center for Particle Astrophysics at the Fermi Laboratory, gives some insight in a recent report. He states that a newly discovered Higgs field "fills all of space and gives particles mass." He goes on to describe it as acting like a "kind of space-filling *molasses*, or that it's like a space-filling crowd of groupies hanging onto a celebrity." Hogan (2012) continues:

Another space-filling field also adds mass to everyday substances, in a way different from the Higgs field. The gluons of the strong nuclear force field create most of the mass of atoms through the energy of their incessant motion inside tiny bubbles of space that we call protons and neutrons. Since the mass-giving gluons are immune to the Higgs field, they have no mass themselves, but only add energy because of their motion. Moreover, they are held inside those bubbles by a gluon field that fills empty space everywhere between the bubbles... in just those places in space where the added mass isn't.

In today's physics, the Higgs boson is thought to confer mass on all the various particles observed. What is significant in this report is the discovery that what gives atoms their mass is "the energy of the incessant motion of the gluons." Gluons are the mediators of the strong force in nature and are considered massless like the photon. So although energy does not occupy much of our thinking in modern-day medicine, it appears to occupy 99.9999% of who we are.

Tiller postulates that *two* (Tiller's emphasis) unique levels of physical reality exist. One is the familiar electric/magnetic dipole, molecular, and atomic states that have been studied by conventional science. The other level of reality appears to function throughout physical space; it interpenetrates the vacuum and the electric/magnetic dipole, atomic, and molecular states. These two states do not usually interact, so one level of reality is invisible to the other and cannot be measured by conventional instruments. Tiller calls this the "uncoupled state" of physical reality. Tiller's research demonstrates, however, that the proper use of human consciousness applied through human intention can cause these two different categories of substances to interact. He refers to this as the "coupled state" of physical reality (Tiller, 2009). Further, Tiller states that "the infrastructure that we build into the many layers of our self via the many aspects of living is a special form of information that increases our level of consciousness and coherence" (personal communication, February 13, 2013). Tiller (2009) concludes:

> Traditional medicine's mindset and working arena is the uncoupled state of physical reality. CAM's working arena is the coupled state. Both sets of practitioners need to become aware of the fact that data gathering strategies that work well for the *uncoupled state* physics do not work well for *coupled state* physics and vice versa.

Tiller's research validates the need to establish different methodologies in researching CAM therapies and practices.

The purpose of this model is not to create a new framework for how the physical and energetic universe operates, but to begin to steer our thinking in a direction that is more inclusive and expansive. One thing is for certain: We are more space than we are matter, and what occupies that space seems to be a dynamic energy. It is only now being appreciated that the dominant energy in our universe does not reside in normal matter or even dark matter of black holes. Rather, it is located in the physical vacuum ("empty space") located between the fundamental particles that make up atoms and molecules (Manek & Tiller, 2012).

As pointed out earlier, it takes a long time to change the prevailing paradigm. The discovery that atoms are mostly empty space was made in 1909 by Ernest Rutherford at Manchester University (Sen, 2007). In spite of this, science has adhered to the materialistic paradigm for more than 100 years. Just as it took Rutherford an enormous amount of courage to report his findings, those of us working in health care will need to be courageous in suggesting a new perspective.

Martha Rogers: A Visionary in Nursing

Martha Rogers's science of unitary human beings is perhaps the most visionary and revolutionary conceptual framework in nursing's history. One of the distinctive characteristics in her framework was how she defined human beings. Rogers created the most expansive and futuristic definition of human beings in nursing's history when she stated that each person is "an irreducible, indivisible, pandimensional energy field identified by pattern and manifesting characteristics that are specific to the whole and which cannot be predicted from knowledge of the parts" (Rogers, 1992, p. 29). Further, Rogers explains that "energy fields are infinite and pandimensional and in continuous motion" (Rogers, 1992, p. 30.). She defined *energy field* as "the fundamental unit of the living and the non-living. Field is a unifying concept. Energy signifies the dynamic nature of the field; a field is in continuous motion and is infinite" (Rogers, 1990, p. 7). The implications of the concepts are far-reaching and help to explain and guide nursing's role in integrative care, especially as it relates to subtle energy therapies and holistic systems of practice.

Rogers provides a definition of who we are that is expansive and can be understood by professionals across disciplines. Rogers perceived the person as an undivided whole. People *are* energy fields; people don't just *have* energy fields. These fields are open and continually in process with other fields. The environment is likewise considered "an irreducible, indivisible, pandimensional energy field identified by pattern and integral with the human field" (Rogers, 1992, p. 29). The person and the environment are both open fields and are both in continual process with each other, which means, from Rogers perspective, that there is no separation. Rogers further explains:

> Unitary human beings are specified to be irreducible wholes.
> A whole cannot be understood when it is reduced to its
> particulars. The use of the term unitary human beings is not
> to be confused with the current popular usage of the term
> holistic, generally signifying a summation of parts, whether
> few or many. The unitary nature of environment is equally ir-
> reducible. The concept of field provides a means of perceiving
> people and their respective environment as irreducible wholes.
> (p. 29)

Rogers changed the word multidimensional to pandimensional to describe energy field. She defines pandimensional as "a non-linear domain without spatial
or temporal attributes" (Rogers, 1992, p. 29). This signifies a domain that is
beyond the time/space continuum and is congruent with the thinking of many
physicists who maintain that the past, present, and future exist simultaneously.
This supports the phenomena of interdimensional beings and energies. This
also creates a theoretical platform for afterlife discussions and can help explain
many paranormal happenings.

Rogers's definitions provide a foundation for an interdisciplinary model that
recognizes the energetic essence of the whole person. Her vision can help
guide us as we move toward embracing a paradigm of health, healing, and
wellness.

Summary

Defining who we are is the first step in developing a model of care. The current
biomedical model cannot explain, predict, or help us understand many of the
phenomena associated with healing or healing therapies. Perceiving ourselves
as simply biological beings is not congruent with concepts in physics that have
emerged over the past century. In addition, the current biomedical model, with

its reductionist perspective, is not effective in dealing with the complexities and interrelated issues involved in chronic disease and health promotion.

This is not to say, however, that the biomedical model is not useful. The biomedical model is useful when studying and intervening in various phenomena occurring within a certain energetic resonance, or the *uncoupled state* of reality (as referred to by Tiller). The present biomedical model is not useful when studying many of the healing therapies and interventions that occur in a more coherent energetic state that Tiller refers to as the *coupled state* of reality. Physics tells us that we are 99.9999% empty space, and that what occupies that space seems to be a dynamic energy. Developing a perspective that acknowledges the energetic and information essence of who we are is important if we are to advance our knowledge and our practices.

Martha Rogers's science of unitary human beings provides definitions and concepts that are expansive and visionary and that can be understood by professionals across disciplines. Her framework has guided much research and knowledge in nursing and can now provide a foundation for an interdisciplinary journey toward health, healing, and wellness.

References

Barrett, E. A. M. (1990). *Visions of Rogers' science based.* New York, N.Y: Nursing National League for Nursing.

Carroll, J. S., & Quijada, M. A. (2004). Redirecting traditional professional values to support safety: Changing organizational culture in health care. *Quality and Safety in Health Care, 13* (Supplement II), ii16–ii21. doi: 10.1136/qshc.2003.009514

Curtis, P. C., & Gaylord, S. A. (2004). Concepts of healing & models of care. In S. Gaylord, S. Norton, & P. Curtis (Eds.), *The convergence of complementary, alternative & conventional health care: Educational resources for health professionals* (pp. 1–26). Chapel Hill, NC: Program on Integrative Medicine, University of North Carolina at Chapel Hill. Retrieved from http://www.med.unc.edu/phyrehab/pim/files/Concepts%20of%20Healing.pdf

Gerber, R. (2001). *Vibrational medicine* (3rd ed.). Rochester, VT: Bear & Company.

Harmon, W. (1998). *Global mind change: The promise of the 21st century* (2nd ed.). Sausalito, CA: Berrett-Koehler Publishers.

Hogan, C. (2012). What fills space? *Fermilab Today* (July 2012 ed.). Fermi National Accelerator Laboratory Office of Science, U.S. Department of Energy. Retrieved from http://www.fnal.gov/ pub/today/archive/archive_2012/today12-07-25.html

Kuhn, T. S. (1996). *The structure of scientific revolutions* (3rd ed.). Chicago, IL: University of Chicago Press.

Lawrence Berkeley National Laboratory. (2012). The particle adventure: Fundamentals of matter and force. U.S. Department of Energy National Laboratory Operated by the University of California. Berkeley, CA. Retrieved from http://particleadventure.org/index.html

Manek, N., & Tiller, W. (2012, April). The sacred Buddha relic tour: For the benefit of all beings. *Toward a science of consciousness conference.* University of Arizona Center for Consciousness Studies, Tucson, AZ. White Paper XXV. Retrieved from www.tiller.org

Reynolds, P. D. (1971). *A primer in theory construction.* New York, NY: Macmillan.

Rogers, M. (1990). Nursing: Science of unitary, irreducible, human beings: Update. In E. A. M. Barrett (Ed.), *Visions of Rogers' science based* (pp. 5–11). New York, N.Y: National League for Nursing.

Rogers, M. (1992). Nursing science and the space age. *Nursing Science Quarterly, 5*(1), 27–34.

Salam, A. (1990). *Unification of fundamental forces: The first 1988 Dirac memorial lecture.* Cambridge, England: Cambridge University Press.

Schein, E. H. (1990). Organizational change. *American Psychologist, 45*(2), 109–119.

Sen, P. (2007). Tiny finding that opened new frontier. BBC news. Retrieved from http://news.bbc.co.uk/2/hi/science/nature/6914175.stm

Tiller, W. (2009). *Why CAM and orthodox medicine have some very different science foundations.* White Paper. www.tiller.org.

3

The Model of Whole-Person Caring: An Overview

"The work is not to introduce a few new ideas, but to change a world view."

–Margaret Wheatley

The model of whole-person caring (WPC) is a framework designed to guide individuals and organizations toward health and wellness. The model operationalizes concepts inherent to healing at both a personal and organizational level. It is an interdisciplinary and holistic model that is derived from theorists in the fields of nursing, physics, and systems theory. It was originally developed to assist health care organizations in creating a healing and nurturing environment for consumers and health care personnel. However, it is equally useful for business, educational, community, and governmental organizations.

This model provides a common framework so that personnel from various disciplines and cultural backgrounds can work together to provide quality care and compassionate service. This contemporary and evolving model will appeal to those individuals and organizations who want to strengthen their workforce and create a sense of meaning and purpose within their culture. The model helps organizations move their vision and mission statements from placards on the wall into the very heart of their operations.

The model of whole-person caring defines who we are from a holistic and more expansive perspective. The model transcends the current paradigm and acknowledges the energetic and spiritual nature of our existence. This viewpoint helps us move beyond our cultural, religious, social, and economic differences and helps us perceive the inherent unity of life. As we begin to see existence as sacred, the way we treat ourselves and each other dramatically changes. Our interactions, work, and relationships begin to arise from a place of deep regard and reverence. This is when true healing begins to occur.

The model provides a way of looking at our world that combines the oldest concepts of nursing and medicine with some of the newest concepts from physics. This is a contemporary and evolving model that will appeal to those individuals and organizations who want to strengthen their workforce and create a sense of meaning and purpose within their culture. This framework will speak to those wanting to infuse their workplace with spirit and soulfulness. The infusion of spirit within the workplace results in an elevated quality of life for everyone—patients and caregivers alike (Pearson, 1999).

The implementation of this model has helped create healthy and healing environments. Programs based on the WPC model have demonstrated the following results:

- Increased health and vitality in participants
- Increased patient satisfaction

- ✿ Increased employee satisfaction

- ✿ Decreased nursing turnover

- ✿ Enhanced communication and teamwork

- ✿ Considerable cost saving

Importance of a Visionary Model

Models help define who we are, what we do, and how we do it. It is important for leaders in health care to begin using models that can fundamentally change how health care is delivered. In the last 4 decades, the health care industry has been driven by business models that embrace the biomedical perspective. Health care has become increasingly unavailable to the greater population, and the delivery of care is often fragmented and impersonal. Creating a system that is more accessible, is less fragmented, and acknowledges our wholeness is not easy.

The primary phenomenon of interest in this interdisciplinary model is how we perceive ourselves as human beings and the implications this has for health and health care organizations. Related concepts include environment, health, whole-person caring, and spirituality. The four concepts of interest to nursing in a model of care include person, environment, health, and nursing (Fawcett, 1993). Because the WPC model is interprofessional, the concept of nursing has been replaced by the concept of whole-person care. The concept of spirituality has also been added because it is foundational to the model. The definitions of person, environment, and health are heavily influenced by concepts put forth in Martha Rogers's science of unitary human beings. The descriptors open, infinite, and mutual process are inherent to Rogers's theory and incorporated into the definitions of person and environment. (See Table 3.1.)

Table 3.1   Concepts and Definitions in the WPC Model

Concept	Definition
Person	An energy field that is open, infinite, and spiritual in essence and in continual mutual process with the environment. Each person manifests unique physical, mental, emotional, and social/relational patterns that are interrelated, inseparable, and continually evolving.
Environment	An energy field beyond and inclusive of the person. Because person and environment are in a state of constant mutual process, there is no distinction from an energetic perspective.
Health	The subjective experience of well-being.
Whole-person caring	The delivery of care and services to promote healing and wellness. Whole-person caring is based on the concepts of the infinite and sacred nature of being, therapeutic partnering, self-compassion, self-care, self-healing, optimal wellness, transformational leadership, and caring as sacred practice.
Spiritual	The spiritual dimension is a unifying field that integrates the physical, mental, emotional, and social/relational aspects of being. The spiritual dimension is the essence of self and transcends the self. It is our closest, most direct experience of the universal life force.

Source: Gold & Thornton, Revised 2013.

Changing the health care system first requires a paradigmatic shift in how we perceive ourselves. How we perceive ourselves and each other dynamically affects how we care for ourselves and each other. As physicists have concluded, the reality of who we are is too rich to be fully expressed in any model or theory. So at best, this model is a metaphor that can help us come to a common understanding or shared perspective of who we are. It is intended to begin to shift the health care community's perception of who we are from being biomedical entities to include the sacred and infinite nature of our being.

The work of three nurse theorists helped form the definition of who we are. As cited by Macrae, Florence Nightingale stated, "We are a reflection of the divine, with physical, metaphysical, and intellectual attributes" (1995). Martha Rogers (1992) saw each person as "an irreducible, indivisible, pandimensional energy field identified by pattern and manifesting characteristics that are specific to the whole and which cannot be predicted from knowledge of the parts" (p. 29). Jean Watson, a contemporary nurse theorist, states, "We are sacred beings [and] we must regard ourselves and others with deepest respect, dignity, mystery, and awe" (personal communication, December 5, 1998).

In the WPC model, the metaphor of a diamond is used to describe who we are. (See Figure 3.1.) As noted in Table 3.1, the model of whole-person caring defines a person as "an energy field that is open, infinite, and spiritual in essence, and in continual mutual process with the environment. Each person manifests unique physical, mental, emotional, and social/relational patterns that are interrelated, inseparable, and continually evolving." In the WPC model, the energy field is considered to be the first field of the manifest universe. It is from this field that all of material existence emerges. Each of us comes from this field, and at this primordial level all of existence is one.

The first manifestation of who we are and the foundation of our being is our spiritual self. Unlike other models that view the spiritual as an aspect of our being, this model purports that the very foundation of our being is spiritual. As Pierre Teilhard de Chardin has said, "We are not physical beings having a spiritual experience, we are spiritual beings having a physical experience" (1965, p. 119).

Arising from this spiritual foundation is the spiritual self, which is the essence of who we are. While this self cannot be seen in Figure 3.1, imagine that it occupies the whole interior of the diamond and is obscured from your view by the physical, emotional, social/relational, and mental facets of existence. When we begin to access and acknowledge our spiritual self, this spiritual essence becomes integrated into each of the facets of our lives and gently transforms us. We begin to realize and understand the sacred nature of our being and move toward self-realization.

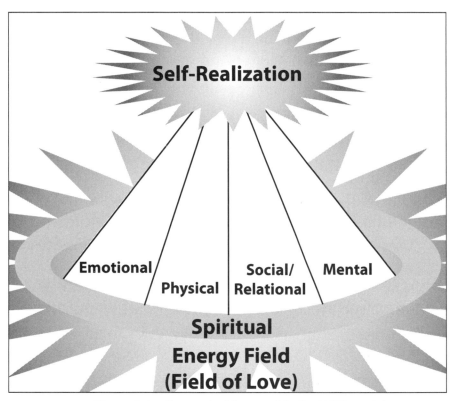

Figure 3.1   Concept of "person" in the WPC model.

The whole-person figure reflects the inseparability of the emotional, physical, social/relational, and mental aspects of who we are. These aspects can be likened to the facets of a diamond. While each facet manifests in a particular way, each remains an inseparable, interrelated aspect of the whole diamond. As Barrett (1994) so aptly said, "In reality, there is no mind, no body, no spirit, only the inherent unity of who we are" (p. 77). Essentially, there are no parts, only facets—or, as Rogers might say, "manifestations" of the whole.

Although this model falls short of expressing reality, it points us in the direction of beginning to understand the implications of our infinite nature. In other words:

> If we are open, infinite energy fields, then not only are we
> finite forms that exist on Earth, but we simultaneously share
> in the essence of the unmanifest Absolute. Also, not only do
> we occupy and move about in our individual physical space,
> but we simultaneously exist in a unified collective energy field
> with all beings. (Thornton, 2003, p. 4)

This model helps us understand what mystics have referred to as "unity" or "cosmic consciousness." The idea that we are all one may seem preposterous in a society that places such high value on individualism and independence. Yet from the perspective of this model, we can see how this can be so. Our sense of who we are, our ego, is contained within the diamond. When our sense of self is dissolved either through extreme trauma, moments of enlightenment, or other peak experiences, our essence, or *higher self*, as it is sometimes called, can perceive the oneness of all that exists. Essentially, the egoic veil has been pierced, and we have been given a glimpse of the inherent wholeness and perfection of the universe.

Importance of an Interdisciplinary Model of Caring

All this may seem hypothetical to someone who is trying to manage a department with an increased workload, increased patient acuity, and decreased numbers of professional staff. One may ask, "What possible relevance does this have to hospital staff, managers, and CEOs?"

First, it is important that an interdisciplinary model be established. The importance of such a model cannot be overstated in an environment in which teamwork and synergy are so important. All the models that exist in health care today focus either on nursing, medicine, or psychology. Establishing a model that provides a common ground for practice is essential in maximizing productivity and creating synergy within the workplace. It will be even more important in the future as health care workers' skill levels and backgrounds become more and more diversified. An interdisciplinary model that can bring people together is important. Such a model has the potential to create a common vision for the future and engage health care members in a common purpose and meaning. According to one management consultant and author, "When aligned around shared values and united in a common vision, ordinary people accomplish extraordinary results" (Blanchard & O'Connor, 1997, p. 7). This is precisely what members of the health care team are being called to achieve: extraordinary results!

Second, an interdisciplinary model is essential in creating the cultural shifts that are important for institutions to remain viable. Most hospitals seek to create an environment that is healing for patients. Increased technology coupled with increasing workloads and decreasing staff create hospital experiences that feel impersonal and uncaring for many patients. According to an organizational consultant, to change the prevailing culture, it is imperative that the movement be all-inclusive and pervasive (Pritchett & Pound, 1993). To change the prevailing biomedical culture toward a culture that embraces healing and caring requires a model that everyone working in the health care setting can understand. An interdisciplinary model provides a common foundation for change to be all-inclusive.

One aspect of this model that makes it particularly useful is its simplicity. The WPC model can be implemented in the hospital or clinical setting and be understood by every staff member and practitioner. In other words, maintenance, housekeeping, administration, trustees, nursing, medical, and ancillary staff can all understand, relate to, and allow their work and decisions to flow from this model. This model can provide the glue that unites the practices and decision-making in an entire organization or health care system.

Inviting Healing Practices and Whole Systems of Medicine into Health Care

The model of whole-person caring is useful in helping to explain the phenomena associated with many healing practices and with whole systems of medicine. By defining who we are as energy fields that are open and infinite in nature, the model creates a framework in which subtle energy therapies—and whole systems of medicine based on subtle energies—make sense. As discussed in Chapter 2, "Redefining Who We Are," many phenomena associated with healing make no sense in the current biomedical paradigm.

Integrating healing therapies into health care practices is useful and often provides cost-effective alternatives to Western medicine. Mind-body-spirit therapies such as prayer, meditation, yoga, affirmations, imagery, and visualization have been effective in a variety of conditions because of their capability to encourage relaxation, improve coping skills, and reduce tension and pain. Massage and other body therapies are useful in reducing anxiety, depression, and musculoskeletal pain. Likewise, subtle energy therapies have been shown to be useful in reducing stress, pain, and anxiety; accelerating healing; and promoting a greater sense of well-being.

Medical systems such as traditional Chinese medicine, Ayurvedic medicine, naturopathy, and homeopathy, which treat the whole person, have valuable contributions to make to our health care system. They focus on prevention, patient empowerment, healthy lifestyles, and the low utilization of high-cost interventions. This places these systems in a position to help shift health care toward a paradigm of health, healing, and wellness that is affordable and sustainable. The model of whole-person caring creates a framework that invites the integration of healing practices and whole systems of medicine. When we perceive ourselves as fields of energy, those practices that are based in modulating and balancing energy systems make perfect sense.

Key Concepts of Whole-Person Caring

The six key concepts of the WPC model are as follows:

- Infinite and sacred nature of being
- Therapeutic partnering
- Self-compassion, self-care, and self-healing
- Optimal wellness
- Transformational health care leadership
- Caring as sacred practice

These concepts serve as the foundation for individual and organizational transformation.

Infinite and Sacred Nature of Being

As mentioned, a key concept in whole-person caring is that it defines people primarily as spiritual (sacred) beings. Both historical and contemporary healers and leaders in nursing have addressed our sacred nature. According to Medieval mystic and healer Hildegard of Bingen, "Man is the work of God, perfected," and everything in nature is a holy temple—an altar for serving God (Flanagan, 1995, p. 149). Florence Nightingale spoke of human beings as a "divine reflections" of God (Macrae, 1995). Jean Watson teaches that the human body is a "sacred temple of the soul" (personal communication, December 5, 1998). When we know that human beings are sacred and deserve to be treated accordingly, our words, actions, and behaviors are significantly affected.

According to Webster's dictionary, the sacred is to be "regarded with reverence" (Webster's, 1989). As we begin to care for those who enter our hospital with reverence rather than as patients with a particular diagnosis, our caring comes from a deep place of love and respect rather than an impersonal place of professional obligation.

Therapeutic Partnering

Therapeutic partnering involves establishing relationships within and among colleagues and clients that promote health and healing. The relationship of partners is nonhierarchical and mutual. Each member of the partnership is regarded with mutual respect, value, and courtesy, and is treated with utmost compassion, admiration, and appreciation (Gold & Thornton, 2000). Table 3.2 compares professional roles in the traditional model of relationships and the model of whole-person caring.

Table 3.2   Comparison of Professional Roles

Traditional Model of Relationships	Model of Whole-Person Caring Relationships
Hierarchical among and within professions	Health care professionals work together as partners in service
Perceived power based on profession, level of service education, and organizational positioning	Concept of power obsolete, replaced by concept of service education, and organizational positioning
Competition and divisive energy are prominent	Mutual support and synergistic energy are dominant
Communication proceeds from top management downward	Communication flows freely between all organizational levels

Source: Gold & Thornton, 2000.

The health care team is composed of numerous partnerships. No department and no team member is more important than another, and every member of the team is crucial in providing the best care possible. The common focus of all professional partnerships is service to the person and the person's family. Every member of the team brings his or her own special expertise and talents. Every profession offers its special focus for care. The common ground of practice is whole-person caring. Each of the disciplines interfaces with the person in different ways, but all converge to provide quality care and compassionate service. In the center of the diamond is the patient, who is at the center of all care and work. Within this framework members of the health care partnership comprise a community of caregivers (Gold & Thornton, 2000), as shown in Figure 3.2.

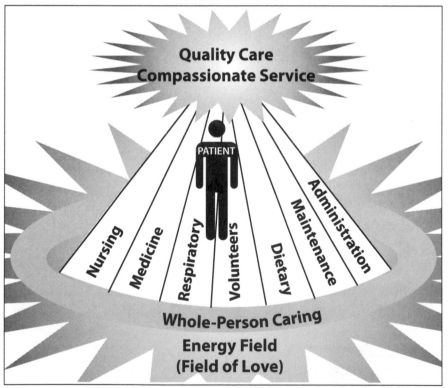

Figure 3.2　Concept of therapeutic partnerships in the WPC model.

The relationship between the person and the health care professional is likewise considered a partnership. The health care professional treats the person with respect and consideration, and plans for care and treatment are mutually established. The health care professional is not an authoritarian figure but a collaborator who brings his or her expertise and skills to the partnership.

Self-Compassion, Self-Care, and Self-Healing

Self-compassion, self-care, and self-healing are primary concepts in the WPC model and are essential in creating a healing culture within the organization. Self-care and self-healing cannot be practiced without an attitude of self-compassion. People must learn to care for themselves before they can care for others. According to one nurse theorist, "We must learn to treat ourselves with love and respect before we are able to treat others that way" (J. Watson, personal communication, December 5, 1998).

Organizations that foster employee participation in wellness programs and offer educational programs on self-care and self-healing help to create a healthier and happier environment. Polls show that half of all Americans say that job stress affects their health, personal relationships, or ability to do their jobs (Hafen, Karren, Frandsen, & Smith, 1996). Offering and encouraging employee participation in exercise/movement classes, yoga, relaxation techniques, meditation, visualization and imagery, and many other approaches are easy ways to involve members of the health care team in caring and healing practices.

Optimal Wellness

Optimal wellness involves all aspects of our being. Within the model of whole-person caring, the spiritual/energetic essence provides the foundation for optimal wellness. It is at this foundational level that unconditional love arises, and our meaning in life and respect for all beings originates. As our spiritual essence is integrated into the various aspects of our life (physical, mental, emotional, and social/relational), patterns of optimal wellness become manifest.

It is important to imagine and know what being well might look like. Most of the focus on wellness is on weight loss, exercise, and nutrition, but in fact, being well involves every aspect of our being. Articulating some of the manifestations of optimal wellness in the different facets of our lives enables us to imagine and visualize ourselves attaining those things. People become so entranced by their habits that they don't take the time to consider alternative possibilities that promote healthier outcomes. Reflecting on some of the manifestations of patterns of optimal wellness can help awaken people to new possibilities. For more information, see Table 8.1 in Chapter 8, "Optimal Wellness."

Transformational Health Care Leadership

Leadership within the model of whole-person caring is transformational in nature. The metaphor of the diamond is used to conceptualize the effect that the WPC model exerts on an organization. Using this metaphor, the organization exhibits its own emotional, physical, social/relational, and mental characteristics. The foundation for leadership is based in the spiritual/energetic realm. The spiritual/energetic field infuses leadership with love, meaning, and respect. In the organization's emotional realm, this manifests as caring, empathetic, and empowering leadership. Leadership arising from spiritual values physically manifests as a flexible, flowing, and vital way of leading. The social/relational aspect reflects a leadership style that is participative in nature and values driven. From the social/relational context, everyone becomes a model of leadership. And finally, from the mental perspective, transformational leadership creates in the organization a strong sense of vision and purpose with a consciousness characterized by awareness and clarity. See Figure 3.3.

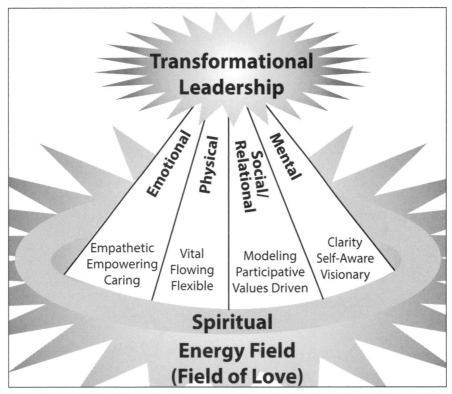

Figure 3.3   Concept of transformational leadership in the WPC model.

Evolving toward transformational leadership is an ongoing process in an organization. Leaders must learn ways of accessing their own spiritual/energetic essence to be effective. Activities and ways of being that can help leaders to access their spiritual nature include prayer, meditation, centering methods, and learning to be fully present to life (Gold & Thornton, 2000). The evolution of leadership is a process of deep inner growth, change, and development. This evolution cannot be directly communicated to others; however, it can be modeled and facilitated by wise leaders. Leadership development is a process of self-discovery and self-appropriated learning (Vaill, 2000). Leadership development within the WPC model is a spiritual process.

Caring as Sacred Practice

Whole-person caring is sacred work. This is because people are sacred beings. Providing health care from this model thus becomes sacred practice (Gold & Thornton, 2000). This is a dramatic shift from the biomedical model, which often views the person as, for example, the triple bypass in room 202. When a health care worker perceives a person as a sacred being, his or her relationship will be much different from the relationship with a person the health care worker perceives primarily in the context of that person's disease process or surgical intervention. Obviously, the health care worker must be proficient in meeting the physical and biomedical needs of the person. However, when interventions are delivered from the whole-person caring perspective, the quality of the relationship changes. Both the person and the health care provider are enriched when actions and interventions arise from a space of caring and unconditional love.

Helping Organizations Meet Current and Future Challenges

The model of whole-person caring is a valuable tool for helping organizations address current and emerging challenges. Attention to spirituality and spiritual values is an important and often neglected component in organizations. Leaders in management are addressing the current lack of meaning and purpose in organizations and encouraging the incorporation of spiritual values as a way to renew workplace morale. The thesis for numerous publications is that major paradigm shifts incorporating spirituality are needed for effective management and renewing vitality in the workplace (Bolman, 1995; Briskin, 1998; Fairholm, 1997; Gallos & Ramsey, 1997; Pauchant, 1995).

In addition, the model of whole-person caring provides an anchor and a stable foundation upon which an organization can operate in times of change and reorganization. Technology, informational databases, operational systems, and health care–delivery systems are changing at ever-accelerating rates. What is hospital protocol today may change tomorrow. Job descriptions, governance, and organizational structures in most health care systems are continually transforming to meet the emerging needs of the populations they serve and to adapt to changes in government and third-party payer reimbursement and regulations. Adopting a health care model that is unchanged by prevailing social and fiscal factors provides organizations with a stable framework to guide their clinical practices and strategic development.

The most compelling reason to adopt the WPC model is to better meet the needs of the health care consumer. The expectations of health care consumers are changing. They are becoming more involved and empowered and are gathering impressive amounts of information from both traditional and non-traditional sources. Consumers feel alienated, uncured, and unhealed by traditional medicine. As a result, they are taking more responsibility for their health and for making their own health care decisions (Thornton & Gold, 1999). The rise in chronic disease demands a multidimensional treatment approach that considers all facets of a person and takes into consideration the interrelatedness of the mental, emotional, physical, and social/relational dimensions. A consumer-driven shift is occurring from a biomedical model of health care to a partnership model of health care (McLeod, 1999). Being treated with respect is increasingly important, and relationship-centered caring and partnership-centered caring are now essential components in quality health care practice (Gold & Thornton, 2000). Table 3.3 contains a comparison of the current biomedical model with the proposed model and shows how the model of whole-person caring is better suited to meet the needs and concerns of the emerging health care consumer.

Table 3.3   Comparison of Models of Health Care Practice

Current Biomedical Model	Model of Whole-Person Caring
People are seen primarily as biological (bio-psycho-social) beings.	People are seen primarily as spiritual (sacred) beings.
Focus is on physical/physiological symptoms and illness.	Focus is on nourishing a person's wholeness (body-mind-heart-soul)
Focus is on diagnosis and treatment of disease.	Focus is on promoting healthy lifestyle practices.
Emphasis is on cure.	Emphasis is on healing/harmony.
Emphasis is on suppression and/or relief of symptoms.	Emphasis is on exploring meaning and source of symptoms.
Illness seen as negative, something to fix.	Illness is seen as an opportunity to explore and shift lifestyle patterns.
The professional is the authority, the one in charge.	The professional is a therapeutic partner.
The professional is emotionally neutral.	The professional's caring is an important component of healing.
The patient is encouraged to rely on the professional for health care needs.	The person is empowered and encouraged to promote his or her own health.
Hierarchical relationships are valued and encouraged.	Nonhierarchical relationships are valued and encouraged; shared governance is the norm.
The professional orchestrates care.	Patient-professional collaboration is welcomed.

Compiled from Thornton & Gold, 1999; Gold &Thornton, 2000;
Thornton & Gold, 2000; Thornton, Gold & Watkins, 2002.

Summary

The model of whole-person caring is an interdisciplinary model that provides a framework to assist health care organizations in creating a healing and nurturing environment for consumers and health care personnel. While originally designed for hospitals, it is equally useful for educational, business, or governmental organizations seeking to improve the health and wellness of their employees and to create a healing workplace environment. Implementation of this model has resulted in increased patient satisfaction, increased employee satisfaction, decreased nursing turnover, increased integration of organizational values by employees, and considerable cost savings.

The model appeals to organizations interested in strengthening the workforce and in creating a sense of meaning and purpose within the workplace. Adopting the model of whole-person caring is a way of bringing spirit back into the workplace. As an organization begins to view its employees and patients as sacred beings, changes begin to occur in every department and every instance of patient contact. Quality care and compassionate service become the standard as each organization customizes and implements the model to fit its particular needs and culture.

The model of whole-person caring creates a framework that invites the integration of healing practices and whole systems of medicine into health care. When we perceive ourselves as fields of energy, practices based in modulating and balancing energy systems make perfect sense. Medical systems such as traditional Chinese medicine, Ayurvedic medicine, naturopathy, and homeopathy, which treat the whole person, have valuable contributions to make to our health care system. They focus on prevention, patient empowerment, healthy lifestyles, and the low utilization of high-cost interventions. The WPC model places these systems in a position to help shift health care toward a paradigm of health, healing, and wellness, and to help provide affordable and sustainable care. Adopting a framework that can explain healing practices and whole systems of medicine is an important first step in their integration into our health care system.

References

Barrett, E. A. M. (1994). Rogerian scientists, artists, revolutionaries. In M. Madrid & E. A .M. Barrett (Eds.), *Rogers' scientific art of nursing practice* (pp. 5–11). New York, NY: National League for Nursing.

Blanchard, K., & O'Connor, M. (1997). *Managing by values.* South Melbourne, Australia: Business and Professional Publishing.

Bolman, L. G. (1995). *Leading with soul: An uncommon journey of spirit.* San Francisco, CA: Jossey-Bass.

Briskin, A. (1998). *The stirring of soul in the workplace.* San Francisco, CA: Berrett-Koehler Publishers.

Fairholm, G. W. (1997). *Capturing the heart of leadership: Spirituality and community in the new American workplace.* West Port, CT: Praeger.

Fawcett, J. (1993). *Analysis and evaluation of nursing theories.* Philadelphia, PA: F. A. Davis Company.

Flanagan, S. (1995). *Hildegard of Bingen: A visionary life.* New York, NY: Routledge Publishers.

Gallos, J. V., & Ramsey, J. (1997). *Teaching diversity: Listening to the soul, speaking from the heart.* San Francisco, CA: Jossey-Bass.

Gold, J., & Thornton, L. (2000). *Creating a healing culture: Whole-person caring.* Roseland, NJ: Gold and Thornton Publishing.

Hafen, B. Q., Karren, K. J., Frandsen, K. J., & Smith, L. N. (1996). *Mind/body health: The effects of attitudes, emotions, and relationships.* Needham Heights, MA: Allyn & Bacon.

Macrae, J. (1995, June). Suggestions for thought from Florence Nightingale: Changing face of healing. *Joint Conference of the American Holistic Medical Association and the American Holistic Nursing Association.* Cassette tape. Phoenix, AZ: Sounds True Recording.

McLeod, B. W. (1999). Relationship-centered care. *IONS Noetic Sciences Review, 48,* 36–42.

Pauchant, T. C. (Ed.). (1995). *In search of meaning: Managing for the health of our organizations, our communities, and the natural world.* San Francisco, CA: Jossey-Bass.

Pearson, C. (1999). Conscious management: Making magic at work. *The Inner Edge.* (Aug/ Sept). p. 4.

Pritchett, P., & Pound, R. (1993). *High velocity culture change: A handbook for managers.* Dallas, TX: Pritchett & Associates.

Rogers, M. (1992). Nursing science and the space age. *Nursing Science Quarterly, 5*(1), 27–34.

Teilhard de Chardin, P. (1965). *Hymn of the universe.* New York, NY: Harper and Row Publishers.

Thornton, L., & Gold, J. (1999). Integrating holism into healthcare for the new millennium. *Surgical Services Management, 5,* 41–44.

Thornton, L., & Gold, J. (2000). The art and science of whole-person caring. *Surgical Services Management, 6*(4), 28–38.

Thornton, L., Gold, J., & Watkins, M. (2002). The art and science of whole-person caring: An interdisciplinary model for health care practice. International Journal for Human Caring 6(2), 38–47.

Thornton, L. (2003). The model of whole-person caring: Re-defining our way. *Bridges,* International Society for the Study of Subtle Energy and Energy Medicine, *14*(2), 1–4.

Vaill, P. (2000). Reflections on time and leadership. *The Inner Edge.* (Dec/Jan) 5–6.

Webster's Encyclopedic Unabridged Dictionary. (1989). New York, NY: Gramercy Books.

4

Integrating the Model of Whole-Person Caring

"The success of the whole system depends on the success of its individual members, while the success of each member depends on the success of the system as a whole."

–Fritjof Capra

Changing the culture of an organization to one that embraces healing and wellness is an enormous endeavor. People have deeply embedded beliefs and values that determine their responses, reactions, and behaviors toward new ideas. Some of these beliefs are not conscious, so individuals may react negatively to situations or new ideas, while having no awareness or understanding of their responses.

Cultures developed in organizations serve as stabilizers to resist change (Schein, 1993). People resist change for several reasons: a reluctance to give up old habits; change may be perceived as a stressor; change involves more work in the short term; and rigid and closed mindsets (Oreg, 2003). So changing a culture is not an easy task. As with most people, health care workers are more skilled at reinforcing the status quo than they are at implementing something new (Appelbaum & Wohl, 2000).

It is important to understand that such a cultural shift takes time, patience, and wise leadership. Maintaining positive outcomes requires continual effort and a sustained vision until values of health and wellness and associated positive behaviors become deeply embedded in individuals and cultures.

Several processes have been identified as factors in successfully integrating the WPC model:

- Assessing the organization's ideology and culture
- Eliciting support from key people
- Involving everyone
- Customizing strategies for implementation
- Honoring and recognizing exemplary people
- Initiating programs for personal growth and transformation
- Incorporating WPC concepts in performance criteria (Thornton & Gold, 2000; Thornton, Gold, & Watkins, 2002; Thornton, 2005)

Assessing the Organization's Ideology and Culture

Any model must be interpreted and expressed in the specific cultural, social, and economic context in which it is implemented and integrated. Identifying the organization's ideology, mission, and values is important in determining whether such a model is congruent with the established culture. How does the WPC model fit into your organization? For instance, a primary focus of this model is that human beings are perceived as spiritual in nature. Can this basic premise be accepted within your hospital or health care system? What are the religious and spiritual beliefs of those with whom you work? How could this model serve as a guide to promote meaning and purpose in people's lives while honoring diverse beliefs? So, the first step in integrating this model is to assess the appropriateness of this model within the context of your particular organization. Elicit the help of other practitioners, staff, and colleagues as you begin your assessment. Talk with fellow employees about how this model could be put into action.

Eliciting Support from Key People

If you determine that the WPC model is appropriate, the next step is to elicit the support of key people in your organization. Involving upper management is crucial for continued success and support. Who within top management holds values and beliefs closest to those proposed in the model of whole-person caring? Is it the CEO, the COO, the director of patient care services, or the director of mission and purpose (if your organization has such a position)? Again, talk with your colleagues and identify those people who already embrace the philosophy of whole-person caring. Which staff members continually demonstrate a caring attitude, leading by applying principles of transformational leadership? Which people within the organization are models of wholesome and healthy living, whose attitudes and work inspire those around them? These are your key people—your core group. Especially important are nurse managers and staff who can model wholesome, healthy, and caring behaviors until these behaviors are embedded in the cultures of each unit.

Involving Everyone

Identifying your core group to spearhead the effort is vitally important. It is essential, however, to involve everyone in the organization. As previously stated, to change the prevailing culture, it is imperative that the movement be all-inclusive and pervasive (Pritchett & Pound, 1993). The model provides a guide and vision of what is possible, but each organization will need to find its own approach and define its own strategies. This is not a short-term intervention; it demands a long-term commitment by employees, management, administration, and governing boards.

Customizing Strategies for Implementation

Organizations can begin in small ways to implement some of these concepts and show their employees that they are valued and cared for. Honoring employees with a special day is a wonderful morale booster and demonstrates that an organization is willing to invest time and money for the welfare of their workforce (Glanz, 1996). Creating ongoing programs to foster the evolution of mature and wise leadership in an organization is of lasting value. One hospital found it effective to designate a nurse on each floor to serve as a model and advisor to other nurses for delivering healing and compassionate patient care. These are nurses who have completed training in transformational leadership and are models of healthy and wholesome behavior. The hospital demonstrates commitment to providing compassionate care by providing extra compensation for nurses serving in this role (N. Moore, personal communication, December 5, 1998).

Executive committees and governing boards need to understand that their continued support is essential for the transformation of the culture. The executive group and directors are responsible for holding the vision for the organization and making the transformation to a healing culture a priority. Including the transformational process as part of the strategic planning and allocating funds to support the initiatives are necessary for the process to be sustainable.

Honoring and Recognizing Exemplary People

It is important to create a way of honoring and identifying exemplary people within the organization. This demonstrates the organization's commitment to reinforcing caring behavior. How can an organization do this? One hospital has identified outstanding personnel by simply including in their patient survey a question such as, "Did anyone provide you with outstanding service during your hospital stay?" The answers the hospital has received have helped administrators identify and give special recognition to personnel whom patients identify as caring and compassionate (J. Lau, personal communication, May 5, 2000).

Initiating Programs for Personal Growth and Transformation

To implement the model of whole-person caring, it is crucial to initiate educational programs that help foster the ongoing growth and transformation of staff members. A key concept of this model involves self-care and self-healing. Therefore, members of the health care team must first learn to care for themselves and develop healthy ways of living and behaving. Utilizing a hospital-based program that can involve a critical mass of hospital employees in personal growth and transformation is important to shift values and create a healing culture within the organization.

Incorporating WPC Concepts in Performance Criteria

Incorporating concepts of whole-person caring into the criteria for evaluating employee performance is a practical way of reinforcing an organization's commitment to caring values. Inviting employees to establish their own evaluation criteria for each job description invests them in the process and increases their commitment to and understanding of whole-person caring. Furthermore, when staff members develop their own evaluation criteria, they establish what is meaningful to them and derive greater satisfaction from their work.

Developing Programs to Facilitate Change

Several programs have been developed to help integrate the concepts of whole-person caring into people's lives and work. These programs have ranged from 1-hour in-services to year-long programs. Organizations determine what their needs are and what format best suits employees' schedules.

One of the first programs that was developed was a "day of renewal." This program introduced nurses and staff to basic concepts of holistic nursing with special focus on self-care and self-healing. These days were usually offered in nurturing, retreat-like settings. This allowed participants time away for reflection and relaxation. An important aspect of this program and subsequent programs was the use of experiential learning. This "day of renewal" program has been recognized for helping to retain nursing staff by improving nurses' ability to cope with stressful situations in the work environment (Nursing Executive Center, 2000). This program has demonstrated its effectiveness in significantly increasing patient satisfaction when offered to a large number of nurses on a medical-surgical floor.

A 2-day program, Creating a Healing Environment, has been very effective in introducing staff to the concepts of whole-person caring. It was designed to explore the concepts of whole-person caring and to help awaken participants to healthy lifestyle practices. Participants are taught skills and provided with tools to enhance their own well-being and to create a healthier work and patient-care environment. This program was designed to create positive changes in the lives of the participants. Much of the learning takes place through inner reflection, experiential exercises, and discussion. All the experiences in this curriculum build upon each other. Participants are first introduced to theoretical concepts that form the basis of the program. Participants are then guided through various aspects of their life and explore what constitutes healthy ways of behaving and living. Each experiential exercise helps participants explore the patterns of their lives, decipher their usefulness, and gain insight into developing healthy and wholesome ways of being. Participants often comment that their lives have been transformed through this program. While each person is affected to differing degrees, participants almost always comment that they feel renewed, refreshed, and revitalized. This new attitude carries into their personal and professional lives.

Programs like these are essential in shifting the culture of the organization to one of health and wellness. When people become healthier, the organization becomes healthier. The programs bring the model of whole-person caring to life in the organization. The model provides the vision, and the programs bring the concepts of caring, healing, health, and wellness into the lives of participants. It is important to offer such programs on an ongoing basis. Developing or acquiring programs that can be offered in-house is useful in supporting and maintaining a healing culture. Regularly offering in-house programs embeds the caring-healing values and WPC model concepts into the organization's operations while decreasing the cost of hiring outside facilitators.

Compatibility with Other Models

The WPC model is compatible with most other models. The WPC model addresses the whole person and as such is broad enough in its perspective to include other models that have more specific focuses. Combining models that are complementary can assist in providing more comprehensive care.

The WPC model is patient centered and relationship focused. As you saw in Figure 3.2 in Chapter 3, "The Model of Whole-Person Caring: An Overview," the patient is at the center of all care and is the focus for all disciplines. Thus, the model of whole-person caring is congruent and complementary to the model of patient- and family-centered care (PFCC). The four core concepts of patient- and family-centered care are respect and dignity, information sharing, participation, and collaboration (The Institute for Patient and Family Centered Care, 2010). These concepts are articulated in the WPC key concepts of sacredness of being and therapeutic partnerships. The PFCC's focus of concern is the patient and family; that model further articulates criteria for establishing, fostering, and nurturing those relationships.

The relationship-based care (RBC) model focuses on relationships: the relationship we have with ourselves (self-care), the relationships we have with coworkers, and the relationships we have with patients and their families. The concepts of therapeutic partnering, sacredness of being, caring as sacred practice, and self-care and self-healing likewise address these relationships.

Jean Watson's theory of human caring, Margaret Newman's theory of health as expanding consciousness, and, of course, Martha Rogers's theory of unitary beings all have concepts that are congruent and foundational with the WPC model.

Using models together can create synergy and amplify the intended results. For instance, using the RBC's commitments to coworkers (see the upcoming sidebar) and other tools specific to the RBC model is a powerful way to enhance some of the teamwork concepts of the WPC model. Combining ideas and concepts from various models can create a custom-designed framework that meets the needs of the organization's culture and patient population. Assessing your organization's ideology and culture is a crucial step in determining the appropriateness of any model.

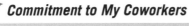

Commitment to My Coworkers

- I will accept responsibility for establishing and maintaining healthy interpersonal relationships with you and every other member of this team.

- I will talk to you promptly if I am having a problem with you. The only time I will discuss it with another person is when I need advice or help in deciding how to communicate with you appropriately.

- I will establish and maintain a relationship of functional trust with you and every other member of this team. My relationships with each of you will be equally respectful, regardless of job title, level of educational preparation, or any other differences that may exist.

- I will not engage in the "3Bs" (Bickering, Back-biting and Blaming) and ask you not to as well.

- I will practice the "3Cs" (Caring, Commitment and Collaboration) in my relationship with you and ask you to do the same with me.

- I will not complain about another team member and ask you not to as well. If I hear you doing so, I will ask you to talk to that person.

- I will accept you as you are today, forgiving past problems, and ask you to do the same with me.

- I will be committed to finding solutions to problems rather than complaining about them or blaming someone for them, and ask you to do the same.

- I will affirm your contribution to the quality of our work.

- I will remember that neither of us is perfect, and that human errors are opportunities not for shame or guilt, but for forgiveness and growth.

–Compiled by Marie Manthey
Reprinted with permission. ©1988, 2013 Creative Health Care Management, Inc.
http://www.chcm.com"www.chcm.com

There may be parts of the model of whole-person caring that are a fit for your organization and other parts that are not. Likewise, there may be aspects of other models that address your needs and some that do not. Ask key people throughout the organization if they think the WPC model is a fit. Whatever is useful, use; whatever is not useful, set aside. Of course, I think the best way to use the WPC model—if the concepts are congruent with your organization—is in its entirety. Each of the concepts supports the others, and when used together, they have a synergistic effect.

The following is a case study by a nurse manager who helped create a healing environment in her hospital using the WPC model (excerpted from Thornton, Gold, & Watkins, 2002).

A Manager's Case Study: The Efficacy of the WPC Model

The model of whole-person caring has been an integral part of creating a healing environment in our health care system. Several years ago, our health care system merged two competing hospitals. A new hospital was built that combined staff from both of the merged facilities. Creating a healing environment in a new hospital that blended staff from two hospitals that were extremely competitive and culturally different was an organizational challenge. The whole-person model of caring helped to create a common ground for the delivery of quality care and compassionate service that transcended the long-standing differences.

Assessing Ideology

The first area that we needed to assess was the congruency between the organization's ideology and the model of whole-person caring. The foundation for our mission statement and values lies in the hospitals' commitment to be of service to our patients and the greater community. Our community places a high priority on spiritual beliefs and feeling connected to the health care that is delivered. The family plays an important role in healing within our small community. The values we use to guide our hospital include respect, honesty, excellence, and teamwork. These same values drive the actions and behaviors of the community we serve. An assessment of the perceived needs of the hospital staff preceded the implementation of the WPC model.

Support from Key People and Establishing a Core Group

Eliciting support from key people was also essential. The director of patient care services, the vice president of patient care services, and the clinical manager leadership group of the hospital were committed to integrating the concepts of whole-person caring. Most importantly, these leaders understood the importance of caring not only for the patients, but also creating ways to support and nurture the hospital employees. The hospital foundation financially supported the educational component of this process as part of our strategic planning.

In addition to administrative support, a core group of nurses was identified to help spearhead the effort throughout the hospital. These were 12 nurses who had completed a holistic course of study and had integrated concepts of self-care and self-healing into their own lives. These nurses served as role models and mentors for other staff.

Involving Everyone

We expanded the number of people who would serve as role models by sponsoring 30 employees to participate in the Certificate Program for Transformational Health Care Leadership (see the section "Initiating Programs for Personal Growth and Transformation").

We also developed a Healing Environment patient care services policy. This policy addresses the importance and expectation that all employees are part of the healing environment and need to be aware and present when in contact with each other and the patient. This includes all disciplines including pharmacy, respiratory, dietary, housekeeping, engineers, nursing, patient registration, etc. Everyone is part of the healing environment, and all are considered healing instruments.

Customizing Strategies for Implementation

We began by offering several "day of renewal" workshops that introduced caring and renewal practices to our staff. These programs were offered in retreat-like settings and provided a time of nurturing, hope, and reflection. The attendees for these days were primarily from the medical-surgical unit of one of our hospitals.

A dramatic increase in patient satisfaction was noted on this particular unit following the days of renewal. This supported our belief that teaching and helping our staff to care for themselves enables them to better care for their patients.

The staff has also initiated many programs that support and foster a healing environment for the hospital and the community. The following are some examples:

- **Programs for health and healing:** Some of the programs that have been staff initiated and staff supported include Parish Nursing, Healing Touch, Massage Therapy, Music Therapy, and the Healing Garden.

- **"On Stage for Healing" concept:** Our hospital floors were designed to separate nursing operations from patient rooms to avoid distractions from the work of healing. Doors divide the patient areas from the backstage area for hospital operations. Signs that say "On Stage for Healing" are placed over doorways as reminders for staff to be fully present and caring as they leave the backstage area and enter the patient-care areas.

- **Spaces and places for healing:** The hospital was designed as a "hospital without walls" to allow for an open and ongoing dialogue with the local community regarding health care needs and the hospital's responsiveness to those needs. The community was invited to participate through a resource library with Internet access and open dining on the first floor mall, where easy locations of services can be found. An interfaith chapel with the parish nurse and chaplain's offices is located proximal to the front entrance, signifying the importance of service founded in spirituality. The outside labyrinth is open to staff and the public 24 hours per day. It includes a pathway of bricks individually dedicated by community and staff members. Trained facilitators offer education and guided walks for the community and the staff.

Honoring and Recognizing Exemplary People

Multiple ways to honor and recognize people and projects have been utilized. Staff members who transformed themselves and their workplace into a healing experience have been featured in the hospital newsletter. The local newspapers published front-page articles on the nursing staff involved in patient care. The hospital foundation magazine published several quarterly articles honoring the transformational staff. The hospital also has an employee-recognition program and identifies employees who receive "values in action" awards from peers and patients.

Initiating Programs for Personal Growth and Transformation

The Certificate Program in Transformational Health Care Leadership was offered over the course of a year to 30 employees. The program provided participants with didactic and experiential teachings that introduced and helped integrate healthy ways of being and coping into their lives and work environments. The program is based on the WPC model and helped familiarize participants with the model's key concepts and ideology. Data collected in a research study to assess the effect of the leadership program supported that the course positively influenced the integration of organizational values among participants. (See Appendix A, "Integration of Organizational Values.")

Quarterly retreats and a bimonthly newsletter were developed to support staff and interested community members in their journey of healing and transformation. Monthly meetings were scheduled outside the hospital for staff to socialize and have fun together. All initiatives were designed to nurture and support the staff in their transformation and to establish the whole-person caring model as the foundation for our healing environment.

Incorporating Whole-Person Caring Concepts into Performance Criteria

On one large, 150-employee unit, the job performance evaluation includes a standard for "Self-Care and Balance." This standard is treated as equally important as the hospital performance standards. In all departments, the guiding values of respect, honesty, teamwork, and excellence are specifically evaluated for each employee.

Summary of Case Study

The WPC model provided a road map for creating a healing environment in our hospital. It helped to shift our paradigm over a 5-year period of time with minimal financial costs. Our nonprofit hospital resides in one of the lowest income-producing counties in Oregon. Our patients and families have, on average, low incomes. We serve a population base that is 65% Medicare.

Progress was steady and resulted in a decrease in turnover of our nursing staff. We believe that the WPC model contributed to employee satisfaction and retention. We experienced a turnover rate of 3% with a full complement of nursing staff after integrating the WPC model. After the WPC model was integrated, there were no open positions in the medical-surgical area, where most of the program development took place. In fact, we needed to create a waiting list for nurses wanting to work in the area.

The roots were fragile and required attention and nurturing as they grew. Just as flowers grow and prosper in their own time, so does our environment as we continually invest in all those who have contact with patients and families to promote healing.

Case Study Results

The WPC model and its associated programs facilitated the creation of a caring and healing culture with quantifiable results. Considerable cost savings were realized as a result of decreased nursing turnover, and patient satisfaction improved significantly. In addition, a research study demonstrated that there was a significant increase in the integration of organizational values in employees participating in the WPC programs. The hospital was the recipient of national, state, and local awards for creating a healing environment and providing compassionate care.

Where Heart and Soul Meet the Bottom Line

The case study attributed significant cost savings to the implementation of the model of whole-person caring and its associated programs in the nursing unit studied. The annual turnover rate dropped to 3% compared to the national nursing turnover rate of 18%. This unit employed 120 full-time nurses; by decreasing their turnover by 15%, they retained 18 more nurses than the national average. They even found it necessary to create a waiting list for nurses requesting to be transferred in. In a 2003 study, the cost of replacing a medical-surgical nurse was estimated to be $92,442. We can extrapolate a savings of $1,663,956 in one year from incorporating the model of whole-person caring (Thornton, 2011).

Increasing Patient Satisfaction

In the hospital studied in the case study, Press-Gainey Patient Satisfaction reports increased to 94% hospitalwide after the model was implemented. Prior to implementation, the average hospitalwide scores were in the low 80th percentile.

After the model was implemented, the hospital was awarded the 2004 Norman Cousins Award. This award, given by the Fetzer Institute, is named for writer and humanitarian Norman Cousins, who, through his life and work, called attention to the importance of relationships to health and healing. The award and its $25,000 prize acknowledges one health care project each year that focuses significantly on relationships.

Creating a work environment that nurtures the heart and soul of its employees and those they serve positively affects the bottom line through nurse retention. Creating a healing environment increases patient satisfaction and positively affects the attitude of the staff. Implementing concepts, practices, and models that improve the quality of care and increase patient satisfaction are more important than ever as reimbursement begins to be linked to positive patient outcomes.

Integrating Organizational Values into the Workplace

A research study showed that employees participating in the Transformational Leadership Course, a program that helps people integrate the concepts of the model of whole-person caring, positively influenced the integration of organizational values. Prior to participation, course participants completed a demographic form and self-report inventory (SRI), which measured the extent to which the respondents had integrated organizational values into their practice. The overall values score, the excellence value, the honesty value, the respect value, and the service value showed a statistically significant increase from pre-test to post-test scores. (See Appendix A.)

Summary

The model of whole-person caring serves as a guide to creating a healthy and healing environment. Creating a culture of healing and wellness takes time, patience, and wise leadership. Some of the steps that have been identified in facilitating a cultural shift are:

- Assessing the organization's ideology and culture
- Eliciting support from key people
- Involving everyone
- Customizing strategies for implementation
- Honoring and recognizing exemplary people
- Initiating programs for personal growth and transformation
- Incorporating whole-person caring concepts in performance criteria

Developing programs that help employees create healthier and more wholesome ways of being are foundational to the success of the organization. To effect change in a person's behavior, the use of experiential techniques such as imagery, visualization, and relaxation techniques are necessary. They help people access both conscious and unconscious patterns of behavior. Offering programs on an ongoing basis is important to continue to reinforce and sustain positive lifestyle changes. Developing or acquiring programs that can be offered in-house is useful in supporting and maintaining a healing culture and decreasing the costs associated with outside consultants and facilitators.

Maintaining positive outcomes requires continual effort and a sustained vision until values of health and wellness become deeply embedded in individuals and cultures. It is important to involve people at every level of the organization in the process of supporting and sustaining the vision. The executive committee and governing board have the responsibility of holding the vision for the organization and making the transformation to a healing culture a priority. Including the transformational process as part of the strategic planning, as well as allocating funds to support the initiatives, is necessary for the process to be sustainable. Especially important are nurse managers and staff who can model wholesome, healthy, and caring behaviors until these behaviors are embedded in the cultures of each unit.

The model of whole-person caring can be used with other models of care such as patient- and family-centered care and relationship-based care. Combining models can create synergy and amplify the intended results.

The implementation of the model of whole-person caring in the case study resulted in savings of over $1.5 million by significantly decreasing nursing turnover. It was instrumental in increasing patient satisfaction from the low 80th percentiles to 94% hospitalwide. A research study showed that the integration of organizational values was increased in employees participating in the model of whole-person caring program.

Implementing concepts, practices, and models that improve the quality of care and increase patient satisfaction are even more important as reimbursement begins to be linked to positive patient outcomes. The most significant and meaningful change that the model helped facilitate was the creation of a healing culture for patients and the staff.

References

Appelbaum, S. H., & Wohl, L. (2000). Transformation or change: Some prescriptions for healthcare organizations. *Managing Service Quality, 10*(5), 279–298.

Glanz, B. A. (1996). Care packages for the workplace: Little things you can do to regenerate spirit at work. New York, NY: McGraw-Hill.

The Institute for Patient and Family Centered Care. (2010). FAQs retrieved from http://www.ipfcc.org/faq.html

Manthey, M. (1988). Commitment to my co-workers. Minneapolis, MN: Creative Health Care Management.

Nursing Executive Center. (2000). Reversing the flight of talent: Practice portfolio. *The Advisory Board.* Washington, DC.

Oreg, S. (2003). Resistance to change: Developing an individual differences measure. *Journal of Applied Psychology, 88*(4), 680–693.

Pritchett, P., & Pound, R. (1993). *High velocity culture change: A handbook for managers.* Dallas, TX: Pritchett & Associates.

Schein, E.H. (1993). How can organizations learn faster? The challenge of entering the green room. *Sloan Management Review, 34*(2), 85–93.

Thornton, L. & Gold, J. (2000). The art and science of whole-person caring. *Surgical Services Management, 6*(11), 28–38.

Thornton, L., Gold, J., & Watkins, M. (2002). The art and science of whole-person caring: An interdisciplinary model for health care practice. *International Journal for Human Caring 6*(2), 38–47.

Thornton, L. (2003). The model of whole-person caring: Re-defining our way. *Bridges,* International Society for the Study of Subtle Energy and Energy Medicine, *14*(2), 1–4.

Thornton, L. (2005), The model of whole-person caring: Creating and sustaining a healing environment. *Holistic Nursing Practice, 19*(3), 106–115.

Thornton, L. (2011). Where heart and soul meet the bottom line: Using the model of whole-person caring to promote health and wellness in your organization. *LOHAS Journal, 12*(1), 31–33.

5

The Infinite and Sacred Nature of Being

"We are not human beings having a spiritual experience, rather we are spiritual beings having a human experience."

–Pierre Teilhard de Chardin

Redefining who we are as human beings is a primary focus of the model of whole-person caring. Broadening our self-perception from biomedical entities to a perspective that acknowledges our spiritual nature is essential. The schism that took place more than 300 years ago between the body, mind, and spirit needs to be bridged. We have neglected our humanity and relegated those things that enliven us, such as love, caring, and compassion, to the backburner.

We are out of balance and need to recover that which we have lost. The dramatic rise in recent years in consumers seeking alternative care is related to a need to be touched and cared for at a more personal level. While today's health care culture is one of brilliant intellectual achievements and remarkable technological advances, spirituality and the human soul have been largely overlooked. Redefining who we are as human beings will not immediately change the way we practice, but it is important that we begin the dialogue.

The dialogue in which we must be engaged is not about abandoning the biomedical model. The questions that must be asked are:

- What is missing?
- What dimensions of ourselves have we left out?
- What is needed to create a system that honors, respects, and creates a compassionate milieu for practitioners and patients?

Is there a place in health care for healing the heart and soul? Or does that remain separate, dealt with in coffee shops and church gatherings? Every hospital and health care system has noble statements about their missions and visions that include respect; trust; caring for the body, mind, and spirit; etc. Is there a way to help organizations integrate their vision and mission statements into the very heart of their operations?

The Human Spirit and Health Care

Acknowledging our spiritual dimension is central to this dialogue. Spirituality is not a new concept in health care; it has been a foundation of practice since the early days of medicine. In the ancient world, medicine and spirituality were intertwined. Healers in temples cared for those suffering with diseases of the body as well as the soul. From the ancient dynasties of China and Middle Eastern kingdoms to the aboriginal empires of the Americas, healing practices were enriched by spiritual inspiration and wisdom, as well as medical knowledge (Ghadirian, n.d.). Florence Nightingale, too, recognized nursing as a spiritual practice. She believed spirituality to be "a driving force in healing…the life principle in humans. It was the thinking, motivating, and feeling part of the human experience" (Dossey, Selanders, Beck, & Attewell, 2005, p. 7).

Accessing our spiritual essence was an important part of healing even in our earliest civilizations. In the last few centuries, however, its importance has diminished as we have responded to the call of technology and materialism. It seems that in many ways, we have lost our connection to ourselves, to nature, and to the very things that enliven us and make us whole.

Differentiating Between Spirituality and Religion

The terms *spirituality* and *religion* are often used interchangeably. While there is definite overlap in these concepts, it is important to differentiate between them. On several occasions when I have been facilitating programs on the WPC model, I have had nurses react negatively to the word *spiritual.* Invariably, when I ask them about their reactions, they express concerns that spirituality represents a viewpoint that will violate their personal religious beliefs. Because the model of whole-person caring considers that the foundation of who we are is spiritual in nature, distinguishing between religiosity and spirituality is important. It is important for people to understand that spirituality is a broad concept that embraces all religious beliefs and honors all people. It does not threaten or question particular belief systems.

A methodological review revealed that agreement exists among nursing and health-related disciplines that spirituality is a broader concept than religiosity and that religion and spirituality are two distinguishable and distinct concepts (Sessanna, Finnell, Underhill, Chang, & Peng, 2011). Conceptual and operational definitions of spirituality and religion vary greatly among nursing and health-related literature. Burkhart and Nagai-Jacobson (2013) provide the following definition of religion:

> Religion refers to an organized system of beliefs regarding the
> cause, purpose, and nature of the universe that is shared by
> a group of people, and the practices, behaviors, worship, and
> ritual associated with that system (p. 721)…Ritual, worship,
> prayer, meditation, style of dress, and dietary observances are
> examples of [religious] practices. (p. 722)

Barnum (2011) states that religion

> no matter what its origin evolves as a social institution…that
> binds people together in many ways. Part of the binding comes
> from shared beliefs, part from communal membership, and part
> from shared rituals. Among its parts, for many members, will
> also be that component we call spirituality. (p. 23)

Religion, then, is a social institution that sometimes—but not always—
includes spirituality. Spirituality, on the other hand, is a personal concept that
can be transcendent, experiential, and existential. Malinsky (2002) helps to
elucidate the differences between spirituality and religion:

> Religion really has little to do with spirituality. Individuals
> may choose to express their spirituality through religion, but
> many spiritual people have no religious affiliation…Spiritual-
> ity is the broader, inclusive term, whereas religion can be nar-
> row and exclusive. Religion is mediated experiencing of the
> sacred; spirituality is direct experiencing of the sacred. Spiri-
> tuality is a unitive experience without boundaries or

divisions. It is about caring for self, others, the natural world, and all that live within it, and about healing. (p. 284)

Hamilton (2010), a neurosurgeon who has written extensively about spiritual phenomena, shares his definition of spirituality:

> I define spirituality very simply as the drive to connect to something greater than ourselves. It is this drive within each of us to reach out to something bigger than just an individual mortal existence. It doesn't matter what you call it; you can call it family, call it consciousness, call it God, or call it nature. I don't care what you call it. I think that has to be part of medicine. It is an inherent part of being. It would be nice to not deny it, but to have a dialogue about it.

Watson maintains that spirituality is one of the most important concepts in our profession and asserts that the care of the soul is the most powerful aspect of the art of caring in nursing (1997). According to Remen (1998), the spiritual cannot be defined as the moral or ethical or religious, stating:

> The spiritual is inclusive. It is the deepest sense of belonging and participation. We all participate in the spiritual at all times, whether we know it or not. There is no place to go to be separated from the spiritual...The most important thing in defining spirit is the recognition that spirit is an essential need of human nature. There is something in all of us that seeks the spiritual. This yearning varies in strength from person to person, but it is always there in everyone. And so healing becomes possible. (p. 64)

In the model of whole-person caring, the spiritual dimension is defined as follows:

> The spiritual dimension is a unifying force that integrates the physical, mental, emotional, and social/relational aspects of being. The spiritual dimension is the essence of self and also transcends the self. It is our closest, most direct experience of the universal life force. (Thornton & Gold, 2000, p. 30)

These examples illustrate the variety of ways that spirituality is expressed. Being an individual concept, the definitions are endless. Personally, I don't like the word *spirituality,* but, as hard as I've tried, I cannot come up with another word that is better. The real difficulty is that what we are attempting to describe is beyond our language. Any description limits that which is essentially limitless. Any one word falls short in attempting to capture the essence of this phenomenal, primal, pandimensional, infinite field of energy and information. Anyone who has ever entered the void or experienced what some call *cosmic consciousness* knows that this space, this level of consciousness, is beyond anything that can be talked about in our ordinary state of awareness. So we are left with a word that cannot be universally defined, that is defined by everyone differently, and from which many people recoil.

Even though we can't define spirituality, most people have come close to it—have felt it, experienced it, and know that it is the power and the force that enlivens us. Whether it's that moment of unity that is experienced on a mountaintop, holding your newborn child for the first time, getting a hole-in-one, being visited by a light being, or seeing the first fruits of one's garden, we have all come close to that feeling of unobstructed love. So although we can't adequately define it, we can dance around and describe what it feels like, how it affects us, and what emotions it engenders within us. And what we notice when we name these attributes is that all the words represent some of our best

qualities and our noblest ideals. Table 5.1 represents some of the attributes
that have been associated with spirituality.

Table 5.1   Attributes Associated with Spirituality

Deep sense of inner knowing	Deep sense of inner peace	Valuing, being valued
Caring, being cared for or about	Equanimity	Hope and harmony
Celebrating life	Deep sense of integrity	Deep sense of gratitude
Compassion for self and others	Being present to life's mysteries	Connected with life's meaning and purpose
Sense of the transcendent	Desire to help others	Forgiveness of self and others
Sense of trust	Giving and receiving love	Sense of well-being
Deep respect for all	Contentment	High level of creativity
Accepting the differences of others	Appreciating beauty or others, the natural world, the universe	Feeling a deep connection with the environment/outdoors

*Compiled from Barnum, 2011; Burkhart & Nagai-Jacobson, 2013;
Sessanna et al., 2011; Thornton, 2012.*

Infinite and Sacred Nature of Being

The model of whole-person caring defines "person" as "an energy field that is
open, infinite, and spiritual in essence and in continual mutual process with
the environment. Each person manifests unique physical, mental, emotional,
and social/relational patterns that are interrelated, inseparable, and continually
evolving." From the perspective of the model, people are infinite and sacred in

nature. This orientation makes a difference in how we approach each other. It shifts how we speak, listen, relate, and interact. When we perceive human beings as sacred, our words, actions, and behaviors are significantly affected.

Moreover, when we view ourselves and others as infinite beings with finite bodies, our relationship to illness, diseases, and death shifts dramatically. Care may be oriented to the soul's purpose in addition to symptom relief. This orientation creates a potential to explore and derive meaning from life's challenges and facilitate healing even in the face of death and terminal illness. Often, nurses have trouble dealing with patients with a terminal illness or who are facing imminent death. When one understands that this physical life is a small part of the infinite journey, the stigma of death becomes obsolete and enables the nurse to be fully present to persons with terminal illnesses and those facing death.

Differentiating Between Healing and Curing

Healing and curing are not the same. Curing is defined as the restoration to health, soundness, or normality and/or the recovery from disease or illness (Cure, n.d.). Curing is primarily involved with the physical. When signs and symptoms of disease and illness are eliminated, we consider a person cured. People often use the terms *curing* and *healing* interchangeably, saying, "I have been *healed* from my cancer, disease, or illness," or, "I have been *cured* of my cancer, disease, or illness."

To heal is defined as "to make sound or whole" and/or "to restore to health" (Heal, n.d.). Both healing and curing are similarly defined as the "restoration to health." Healing however, is a much broader concept, also concerned with "making sound or returning to wholeness." The process of returning to wholeness is one that can involve every aspect of our being. Any part of our lives that are broken, any aspect of our being that is wounded, can be made whole through healing. Malinsky (2002) writes:

> Healing is the creative potential continuously flowing throughout the universe. Healing involves being aware of, sensitive to, and cherishing wholeness for self, others, and the environment apart from disease conditions, traumatic situations, or the like. Cure may not be possible in all situations, but healing is the potential in all situations. (p. 284)

Healing, then, is not synonymous with cure and recovery. Healing may occur at any time, independent from illness or disease. A person may experience healing in the process of dying—for example, after reconciling a long estrangement from a family member. People who are chronically ill may experience healing as they learn to accept their limitations with equanimity rather than anger and bitterness. Often, healing involves restoring meaning and purpose to our lives.

Apollonius of Tyana, the most famous philosopher of the Greek-Roman world of the first century, recorded Pythagoras as saying:

> [T]he most divine art was that of healing. And if the healing art is most divine, it must occupy itself with the soul as well as with the body; for no creature can be sound so long as the higher part in it is sickly. (Mead, 1901)

The soul, the higher part of us, our spiritual self, was a vital force and an integral dimension of health and well-being in the worldview of early healers. For the past 300 years, however, health care has been primarily involved with the treatment of illness and disease, and has excluded this primal energetic ground of being that gives meaning and purpose to our lives. We have occupied ourselves primarily with curing. It is time to rediscover our role as healers. To do so, we must acknowledge and embrace the sacred and infinite nature of our being.

Creating a Healing Environment: Integrating Spirituality into the Workplace

What are some steps that can help us integrate spirituality into the workplace? How do we create a healing environment for ourselves, our colleagues, and those we serve? I have identified several steps and approaches that are useful to support the integration of spirituality into the workplace. (Every organization is different, so remember these are only guidelines.)

- Setting the intention, creating the vision, and beginning the dialogue
- Creating reminders for staff, patients, and families
- Creating healing spaces for patients, families, and staff
- Developing policies to support healing environments
- Developing and mentoring staff

Setting the Intention, Creating the Vision, and Beginning the Dialogue

The core group sets the intention and creates a vision for what they want to manifest. As mentioned in Chapter 4, "Integrating the Model of Whole-Person Caring," developing a core group to help champion the WPC model is important. Usually, the champions for creating a caring and healing environment are the chief nursing officers, nursing managers, or staff nurses. Several hospitals have had physicians either on staff or in administrative positions who have championed the effort in their hospitals, and some CEOs have also led the effort. Involving people from all aspects and levels of the organization is ideal. As mentioned, it is imperative to involve everyone in some way so that creating a caring and healing environment can become a part of each person's vision.

Beginning the dialogue on spirituality should take place at every level. If someone in upper management or on the governing board is in your core group, then that person needs to initiate the dialogue with the executive committee and the board. How this is done depends on the dynamics of each organization. It may involve a simple presentation or suggesting that the mission statement be reevaluated to include words like *spiritual, caring,* and *healing* (if it does not already). Engaging the group and beginning the dialogue is the goal. Concepts like spirituality are difficult for many people to understand, especially those who are focused on the material and concrete aspects of life. People involved in the business and financial aspects of the organization often are unable to relate to abstract concepts. Talking about the money that will be saved by reducing staff turnover and by increasing patient satisfaction will help to engage this group in the dialogue.

Initiating the dialogue on spirituality with employees is most important. Sending out a short survey asking employees to describe their current work environment and how they would change it to create a healing environment for themselves and their patients is an easy way to solicit input. This gets staff involved in the process and invites them to begin thinking about creating a healing environment, as well as encourages them to examine their ideas about spirituality. It also lets staff know that the organization values their input and is interested in creating a caring and healing milieu.

Holding focus groups and inviting employees to contribute their ideas will further energize the process. The more you can engage the staff and the greater their input, the better your results. Also, if you hold focus groups, you will have an opportunity to identify issues that are of concern to employees that can be incorporated into your programs later on. If your organization has unit governance committees in place, this is an obvious place to solicit input.

Remember, growing a caring-healing organization that will be sustainable is an organic process. So proceed through all the processes with patience, respect, and a caring and healing attitude. In doing so, you will be modeling the very behaviors you want to manifest in your organization.

Creating Reminders for Staff, Patients, and Families

Reminders are little things that refocus attention on the goal of creating a healing environment. Displaying a reminder in the form of a poster is easy and effective. Soliciting input from staff works well in this process. Asking staff to contribute a statement of their own vision for the type of care they intend to deliver or the type of environment they want to create will involve them in the process. A graphic designer can create posters with a single statement or a collage of statements that can be displayed in hallways, family waiting areas, and break rooms.

The "On Stage for Healing" signs mentioned in the case study in Chapter 4 are an excellent example of reminders that can be easily implemented. These signs were placed above the exit doors of the staff rooms leading into the patient areas. The signs remind staff to set aside their own concerns and focus on their role as healers as they enter the patient areas.

Including a "Caring/Healing" column in your hospital newsletter or e-news that focuses on a concept of spirituality and recognizes employees and management for their contributions is easy and reinforcing. The newsletter can highlight acts of kindness and include inspirational stories, quotes, or poems.

One hospital put Appreciation Boxes on each of its floors. These were used by patients and families to acknowledge special care they received from any employee. Pins with hearts were given to employees; every time the employee was acknowledged by a patient, he or she was given a colorful bead to add to his or her pin.

These are just a few examples. Again, involving staff, administration, and management in creating their own reminders is a useful process. You will be both delighted and surprised by the wonderful ideas and suggestions that people in your organization will contribute as they become more and more involved in creating a healing environment.

Creating Healing Spaces for Patients, Family, and Staff

Most organizations do not have the luxury of building or remodeling a facility. However, there are simple things that can be done to create a healing environment. Some ideas include the following:

- Incorporating pictures with soothing natural landscapes and other artwork
- Using color in rooms and hallways
- Removing clutter in stock rooms
- Creating employee and family break rooms that are comfortable and calming

Providing soothing music or healing videos, creating gardens or communal areas where people can gather, and creating more sources of natural or full-spectrum light are just a few other ideas.

TIP

Many architectural firms specialize in creating healing environments. If your hospital is considering building new facilities or remodeling, it would be useful to hire a consulting firm or architect that specializes in this area.

In one hospital, several nurses got together over a weekend and transformed their break room with color, incorporating comfortable chairs and a table that they bought at a garage sale. It needn't be an expensive undertaking; much can be accomplished with staff involvement and some discretionary funds.

Developing Policies to Support Healing Environments

It is useful to create a policy on maintaining a healing environment. This policy can identify caring and healing behaviors that are expected from employees and identify negative behaviors that will not be tolerated. Addressing specific behaviors that promote therapeutic and healing relationships helps to clarify expectations and set the intention of creating a healing environment.

Another useful policy is one that supports holistic nursing in the hospital. This reinforces the organization's intention and commitment to providing whole-person care. Holistic nursing is recognized as a nursing specialty by the American Nurses Association (ANA); the American Holistic Nurses Certification Corporation offers several levels of national board certification. Supporting nurses in the process of board certification is another way to demonstrate a commitment to whole-person care.

Finally, developing a policy that addresses the use of healing practices in the hospital will further support a healing environment for patients and staff. Some of the most common therapies available to patients in hospitals, in the order of the frequency of their usage, include the following (Samueli Institute, 2007):

- Pet therapy
- Massage therapy
- Music therapy
- Guided imagery
- Acupuncture
- Biofeedback
- Meditation
- Therapeutic touch or healing touch
- Aromatherapy
- Art therapy
- Chiropractic care
- Hypnosis
- Reiki
- Reflexology

Developing and Mentoring Staff

The process of staff development and mentoring is ongoing. Identifying staff members who can serve as role models for other staff members on each floor helps sustain and reinforce a culture of healing. As mentioned, one hospital has incorporated this idea, providing extra compensation for the nurse serving as a mentor. Role models are staff members who possess many of the spiritual attributes and have been engaged in their growth and development over the years. Finding a staff person who is familiar with healing practices, and who can facilitate training sessions for others, would be ideal.

Because of the need for ongoing programs, it is useful if in-house educators and facilitators can be trained to conduct seminars and workshops for hospital staff. The type of educational program that supports a healing environment must be experiential in nature to facilitate personal transformation. Our spiritual nature is our deepest sense of self; if we want to cultivate that, we must engage in experiential activities that can access that dimension.

A 2-day program associated with the model of whole-person caring has been useful in introducing staff to the WPC model. Hospitals that have incorporated the model find this program to be useful in jump-starting the process. The program is based on each of the concepts of the model: sacredness of being, self-care and self-healing, optimal wellness, therapeutic partnering, transformational leadership, and caring as sacred practice. The program is designed to promote growth through didactic and experiential exercises that increase self-awareness and self-compassion. The self-care and self-healing practices that participants learn in the program can be utilized for their own wellness plan as well as to teach patients. Participants explore every aspect of their lives through introspection, guided imagery, and relaxation. In addition, the program addresses issues related to effective communication, teamwork, and creating therapeutic relationships.

If a critical mass of employees can embrace healthy and wholesome ways of being, behaving, and relating, then the whole organization will soon be transformed. The percentage of people needed to achieve a critical mass is roughly 10%, although some people say it can be as low as 3% or 4%. Creating a plan that allows a critical mass of staff to attend programs that will introduce them to the WPC concepts will support the cultural shift toward a healthy, healing, and caring environment. In-services are needed on a regular basis to reinforce concepts and keep employees engaged. Using motivational and instructional media is an easy way to reinforce concepts and behaviors without creating additional demands on staffing.

Summary

Redefining who we are as human beings is a primary focus of the model of whole-person caring. Broadening our view from perceiving ourselves as biomedical entities to a perspective that acknowledges our sacred and infinite nature is essential. Although today's health care culture is one of brilliant intellectual achievements and technological advances, spirituality and the human soul have been largely overlooked.

As health care workers, we must begin a dialogue—not one that focuses on abandoning the biomedical model but one that asks, what is missing and what dimensions of ourselves have we left out of our care? Spirituality is central to this discussion and central to creating a caring and healing environment.

Differentiating between spirituality and religion is important. Religion refers to an organized system of beliefs shared by a group of people. It is a social institution that often, but not always, includes spirituality. Spirituality, on the other hand, is a personal concept; as such, it is defined in many ways, depending on a person's experience and expression of spirituality. The WPC model defines the spiritual dimension as a "unifying force that integrates the physical, mental, emotional, and social/relational aspects of being. The spiritual dimension is the essence of self and also transcends the self. It is our closest, most direct experience of the universal life force."

Viewing ourselves as infinite and sacred beings changes our relationship to illness, disease, and death. Care may be oriented to the soul's purpose in addition to symptom relief. This orientation creates a potential to explore and derive meaning from life's challenges and to create a healing environment even in the face of death and terminal illness.

Healing and curing are different processes. Both healing and curing are defined as "restoring the body to heath." Although curing is mainly concerned with the physical, healing is a multidimensional process that can involve the body, mind, heart, and spirit. Healing can occur without curing and often involves a spiritual component that helps restore a person's wholeness. Our health care system has primarily been concerned with curing. Rediscovering our role as healers is important in caring for the whole person.

Several steps are useful in integrating spirituality into the workplace:

- Setting the intention, creating the vision, and beginning the dialogue
- Creating reminders
- Creating healing spaces
- Developing policies
- Developing and mentoring staff

These steps are just suggestions; every organization will evolve its own process. The primary force for creating and sustaining a healing environment lies in the development of the staff. Staff development is an ongoing effort, so training in-house staff to become facilitators and leaders for programs, workshops, and in-services is desirable and financially prudent.

References

Barnum, B. S. (2011). *Spirituality in nursing: The challenges of complexity* (3rd ed.). New York, NY: Springer Publishing.

Burkhart, M., & Nagai-Jacobson, M. G. (2013). Spirituality and health. In B. Dossey & L. Keegan (Eds.), *Holistic nursing: A hand-book for practice* (6th ed.) (pp. 721–749). Sudbury, MA: Jones & Bartlett.

Cure. (n.d.). In *Merriam-Webster's online dictionary* (11th ed.). Retrieved from http://www.merriam-webster.com/dictionary/cure

Dossey, B. M., Selanders, L., Beck, D. M., & Attewell, A. (2005). *Florence Nightingale today: Healing leadership global action.* Silver Spring, MD: American Nurses Association.

Ghadirian, A. M. (n.d.). Dr. Abdu'l-Missagh Ghadirian's homepage. Retrieved from http://www.medicineandspirituality.com/index.htm

Hamilton, A. (2010). Bridging medicine and spirituality: An interview with Dr. Alan Hamilton. Superconsciousness: The Voice for Human Potential. Retrieved from http://www.superconsciousness.com/topics/knowledge/bridging-medicine-and-spirituality

Heal. (n.d.). In *Merriam-Webster's online dictionary* (11th ed.). Retrieved from http://www.merriam-webster.com/dictionary/heal

Malinsky, V. (2002). Developing a nursing perspective on spirituality and healing. *Nursing Science Quarterly, 15*(4), 281–287.

Mead, G. R. S. (1901). *The philosopher explorer and social reformer of the first century AD.* Retrieved from http://gnosis.org/library/grs-mead/apollonius/apollonius_mead_16.htm

Remen, R. (1998). On defining spirit. *The Institute of Noetic Sciences Review: 25th Anniversary Issue, 47,* 64.

Samueli Institute. (2007). Survey of Healing Environments in American Hospitals: Nature and Prevalence. Alexandria, VA. Retrieved from http://www.samueliinstitute.org/File%20Library/Our%20Research/OHE/Reportwithinstrument9-18.pdf

Sessanna, L., Finnell, D. S., Underhill, M., Chang, Y., & Peng, H. (2011). Measures assessing spirituality as more than religiosity : A methodological review of nursing and health-related literature. *Journal of Advanced Nursing, 67*(8), 1677–1694.

Teilhard de Chardin, P. (1965). *Hymn of the universe.* New York, NY: Harper and Row Publishers.

Thornton, L., & Gold. J. (2000). The art and science of whole-person caring. *Surgical Services Management, (6)*11, 28–38.

Thornton, L. (2012). *Creating a healing environment: For ourselves, our patients and our co-workers.* Fresno, CA: Seminar Manual.

Watson, J. (1997). Artistry of caring: Heart and soul of nursing. In D. Marks-Maran & P. Rose (Eds.), *Nursing: Beyond art and sciences* (pp. 54–62). Boulder, CO: Colorado Associated University Press.

6

Self-Compassion, Self-Care, and Self-Healing

"The moment you see how important it is to love yourself, you will stop making others suffer."

—Thich Nhat Hanh

Self-compassion, self-care, and self-healing are key concepts in the model of whole-person caring. Self-care and self-healing cannot be practiced without an attitude of self-compassion.

In facilitating a shift toward healing and wellness, it is important to become aware of the underlying dynamics that keep us from changing. Why are some behaviors so hard to change? What keeps us stuck in unhealthy patterns of living? As mentioned, some of the reasons people resist change include the following (Oreg, 2003):

- People are reluctant to give up old habits.

- Change is perceived as a stressor.

- Change involves more work in the short term.

- People have rigid and closed mindsets.

Frequently, however, a deeper dynamic is at work, which keeps us from creating healthier ways of being. Often, we have a fundamental attitude—either conscious or unconscious—that we are not worthy of treating ourselves well or being loved.

Tara Brach, a clinical psychologist and meditation teacher, developed the phrase "the trance of unworthiness" to describe this perception (2004). This trance is characterized by feelings of inadequacy and insufficiency that can be triggered at any moment by a subtle criticism, an argument, a less-than-perfect evaluation—the list is endless. This underlying attitude of unworthiness frequently keeps us from moving forward in our lives. This lack of compassion toward ourselves can impede our progress and keep us from making self-care a regular part of our lives.

Components of Self-Compassion

Within the last decade, self-compassion—a concept that was first taught as part of the Buddhist tradition—has been identified as an important construct in self-care and wellness. According to Neff, self-compassion involves three basic components:

- Self-kindness versus self-judgment

- A sense of common humanity versus isolation

- Mindfulness versus over-identification

These components combine to create a self-compassionate frame of mind (Neff, 2003, 2009).

Self-Kindness Versus Self-Judgment

Self-compassion involves opening your heart to yourself. It invites you to be kind, gentle, and loving toward yourself. Self-compassion is not narcissistic, nor does it inflate your ego. It involves treating yourself with tenderness and understanding. This is in contrast to criticizing or harshly judging. How do you respond when you have fallen short of your expectations, overeaten, or had an angry outburst? Do you use harsh language and demean yourself? Do you disassociate and eat the rest of the box of chocolates? Or, do you look upon yourself through the eyes of a wise grandmother who understands that imperfection is part of the human experience, and who loves and accepts you just as you are?

Letting go of perfection and unrealistic expectations that we have held for a lifetime is not easy. Being understanding with ourselves rather than being harsh and judgmental are habits that take time to alter. A daily meditative practice that can help bring self-compassion into your life is the loving-kindness meditation, discussed in the upcoming sidebar. There are many variations of the loving-kindness meditation. (See Appendix B, "Loving-Kindness Meditation for Beginners.") With any interior practice, the important thing is to do what is comfortable for you and what resonates with your heart and soul. Take time to explore and create a practice that works for you.

Loving-Kindness Meditation

This meditation is a 2,500-year-old practice that uses repeated phrases, images, and feelings to create loving-kindness and compassion toward oneself and others. You can begin by repeating the phrase for 10 to 20 minutes each day. There are many variations of the verses. Feel free to modify the meditation in any way that resonates more deeply with you. The verse below is taught by meditation teacher Jack Kornfield (1993):

1. Sit quietly in a comfortable position. Scan your entire body for any areas that might be carrying tension and gently stretch and move your body in ways that release that tension.

2. Set aside any concerns or worries—you can pick them up at the end of the meditation.

3. Bring to mind a person, place, or thing that evokes a loving feeling within you. It may be holding a newborn baby, hugging a loved one, cuddling your pet, or being caressed by the sun on a sandy beach.

4. Let your consciousness rest in that feeling of love, and with each inhalation imagine that you are infusing your body with a golden light that feels warm and loving. With each exhalation, imagine that you are ridding yourself of any negative thoughts or feelings. Continue this process for several breaths or until you feel relaxed.

5. Inwardly recite the following verses to yourself. Pause and experience the "feeling" of each sentence before proceeding to the next.

   May I be filled with loving-kindness.

   May I be well.

   May I be peaceful and at ease.

   May I be happy.

   Repeat the phrases over and over, allowing the feelings to permeate your body, mind, and emotional being. Observe and acknowledge any thoughts that are distracting or irritating and simply return to repeating the verse. Continue this practice for several weeks, and when you feel ready you can expand the focus of your loving-kindness to include others.

Source: Thornton, 2011, p. 45; 2013, p. 36.

A Sense of Common Humanity Versus Isolation

It is common when we are suffering to feel that we are the only ones experiencing such difficulty. This creates a sense of isolation and loneliness that further contributes to our suffering. By understanding that the suffering we experience from misfortune or mistakes is universal, we begin to feel more compassionate toward ourselves. And when we see our experience as part of the larger human experience, we begin to have deep feelings of compassion for ourselves and others.

Mindfulness Versus Over-Identification

The third component of self-compassion is the ability to hold our painful thoughts and feelings in balanced awareness. Simply put, this means that you do not get too wrapped up in your feelings. Mindfulness involves an open and receptive attention to and awareness of what is occurring in the present moment. Incorporating mindfulness practices allows you to take a step back and observe what is happening and not over-identify with the feelings that you are experiencing. Engaging your observer, discussed in the upcoming sidebar, is a mindfulness technique that enables you to observe what is happening and helps you respond to a situation with equanimity rather than harsh judgment and over-identification.

Over-identification occurs when we become overly focused or fixated on negative thoughts or emotions. In stressful situations, when we are engulfed by negative feelings, our awareness narrows and we cannot perceive things clearly. Mindfulness practices help neutralize the negative reactions and enable us to pay attention and be present to what is happening. Sometimes, even a deep breath or two accompanied by an affirmation such as, "I am at peace, I am present to the moment," allows us to disconnect from the negative feelings so that our vision and thinking can become clearer.

Engaging Your Observer

Engaging your observer is a helpful process when confronting difficult situations, thoughts, or feelings. The *observer* or *witness* is simply the wise and nonjudgmental aspect of yourself. The observer can be likened to a wise grandparent who looks sensibly upon the thoughts and reactions of our childlike minds. It gives us the ability to observe life without engaging our past patterns and reacting emotionally. The *observer* acts as a third party that allows us to separate from personal feelings so that our perceptions arise from a space of clarity and wisdom. Using this technique enhances self-knowledge and self-awareness as it provides constant feedback related to our responses and reactions to situations. Engaging your observer involves centering yourself, being aware of internal reactions, acknowledging these reactions, and responding from a place of wisdom and compassion.

Steps Involved with Engaging Your Observer

Situation: You just realized that you gave your patient the wrong medication.

- **Center yourself:** Take a deep breath, bring your attention to the area around your heart, and connect with a feeling of love and compassion. You might imagine holding a newborn baby, hugging a loved one, or cuddling your pet.

- **Observer relates your internal reactions emotionally, mentally, and physically:** This makes you feel horrible. You are upset that you made this mistake. You are concerned about your patient, what your supervisor will say, and filling out an incident report. Your stomach is upset, and you feel like crying.

- **Acknowledge your reactions:** Yes, I feel horrible when I make mistakes, and I am concerned about the patient, my supervisor's response, and having to fill out an incident report. My stomach hurts, and I feel like crying.

- **Respond from a place of wisdom and compassion:** Take another deep breath, bring your attention to the area around your heart, connect with a feeling of love and compassion, and respond silently to yourself with a self-compassionate remark: Making mistakes is part of being human. Don't be so hard on yourself. This is a great opportunity to learn and grow and become a better nurse.

Source: Thornton, 2008, p. 47; 2011, p. 43.

Identifying what may be blocking us from feeling love and compassion toward ourselves is an important first step. What is it that keeps us in this trance of unworthiness? Some lay blame on the values of our Western culture, which encourage competition, getting ahead, having the perfect body, or having to prove your worth to fit in, to name a few. Others attribute the inability to be self-compassionate to early childhood experiences, trauma, and parental patterns. Research indicates that *greater* self-compassion is associated with those individuals who experienced compassionate parenting. Conversely, *decreased* self-compassion is associated with parents who were critical and judgmental (Neff & McGeehee, 2010).

The primary intention of the WPC model is to help us redefine who we are and to awaken to our true nature. Regardless of what may have caused our unworthiness trance, it is important to realize and embrace our sacred nature. Awakening to our true nature and understanding that we *are precious beings* helps to dispel this trance and allow self-compassion and love into our lives. Learning to be compassionate toward ourselves is a lifelong process. It is a process that we engage in every moment as we open our heart in the face of life's difficulties and embrace an attitude of kindness toward ourselves. There are various practices that can help us develop compassion toward ourselves and others, including the meditation described in the upcoming sidebar.

Breathing Compassion In and Out

This meditation is derived from the Tibetan practice of giving and taking (*tonglen*). In that meditation, the practitioner inhales the pain and suffering of another individual and exhales kindness and compassion. This process subtly reverses our instinctive tendency to resist or avoid emotional discomfort, which usually leads to greater suffering.

This meditation, breathing compassion in and out, adds the medicine of compassion to each inhalation. This meditation can be practiced formally or informally throughout the day for any length of time.

1. Sit comfortably, close your eyes, and take a few relaxing breaths.

2. Scan your body for physical stress, noting the location and quality of the discomfort. Also allow yourself to become aware of any stressful emotions that you may be holding in your field of awareness. If a challenging person comes to mind, let yourself be aware of the stress associated with that person. If you are experiencing the suffering of another person through empathy, let yourself be aware of that discomfort as well.

3. Now, aware of the stress you are carrying in your body, inhale fully and deeply, drawing compassion inside your body and filling every cell in your body with compassion. Let yourself be soothed by inhaling deeply and by giving yourself the compassion you deserve when you experience discomfort.

4. As you exhale, send out compassion to the person who is associated with your discomfort, or exhale compassion to living beings in general.

5. Continue breathing compassion in and out. Occasionally scan your inner landscape for any distress and respond by inhaling compassion for yourself and exhaling compassion for those who need it.

6. Gently open your eyes.

Source: Germer, 2013.

The Importance of Self-Compassion

There are a variety of reasons that self-compassion is important. One of the primary reasons is that you must be able to treat yourself with compassion before you can be compassionate toward others. Healthy compassion occurs when you have learned to honor your own needs and are able to set boundaries and limits. When you can accept yourself, love yourself, and treat yourself kindly in spite of your shortcomings, then you can treat others that way. Your compassion arises from a place of deep authenticity; with it, you become a potent force of healing in this world.

Practicing self-compassion also helps prevent burnout and compassion fatigue. When you listen to and honor your own needs, you are less likely to overextend and exhaust yourself. When you learn to care for others, yet not get entangled in or over-identify with their suffering, your compassion will be less fatiguing.

When genuine compassion and wisdom come together, we honor, love, praise, and include both ourselves and others. Instead of holding the ideal that we should be able to give endlessly with compassion for all beings "except me," we find compassion for all beings including ourselves. The separation of self and others melts away. Then, like the sun rising, the strength of generosity and compassion grows in our practice, and we discover it to be our true nature (Kornfield, 1993).

Research shows that self-compassion is linked to greater emotional resilience and psychological well-being. One of the most compelling and consistent findings is that greater self-compassion is linked to less anxiety and depression (Neff, 2003; Neff, Hseih, & Dejitthirat, 2005; Neff, Kirkpatrick, & Rude, 2007; Neff, Pisitsungkagarn, & Hseih, 2008). In addition, self-compassion is strongly associated with emotional intelligence and wisdom. Self-compassionate people are happier, have better emotional coping skills, and feel more connected to others. Less afraid of failure, they tend to be more intrinsically motivated to learn and grow (Neff, 2009). The increased coping skills and emotional resilience and the decreased anxiety and depression associated with self-compassion make this practice essential.

Concepts of Self-Care and Self-Healing

Self-care and self-healing are foundational concepts in the WPC model. Caring for ourselves involves every aspect of our being. It entails caring for our body, mind, heart, and soul. Self-care and self-healing practices help us live a more balanced life and facilitate greater health, harmony, and productivity. The healthier and more balanced we are, the more effective we'll be in helping and caring for others.

Self-care and self-healing practices are not two distinct categories of practice but are interchangeable. For instance, the American Holistic Nurses Association (AHNA) identifies the following as self-care activities: exercise, grooming, massage, yoga, conscious eating, quiet contemplation, healthy breathing, meditation, healing music, laughter, prayer, and inspirational reading (n.d.). Briggs (2010) provides the following list of self-healing practices: yoga, tai chi, qigong, massage, meditation, aromatherapy, herbal support, nutritional support, music therapy, visualization, prayer, breathing techniques, and reflexology. The overlap is considerable. The lists, while representing only a fraction of possible practices, demonstrate little differentiation between self-care and self-healing practices.

Self-care involves activities to restore and promote health, prevent disease, and limit illness. As mentioned, practices involved in self-care are often interchangeable with those involved in self-healing. For instance, meditation can improve our health by decreasing blood pressure and reducing anxiety, and it can also bring us closer to our spiritual essence.

The World Health Organization defines self-care as follows (1984):

> Activities individuals, families, and communities undertake
> with the intention of enhancing health, preventing disease,
> limiting illness, and restoring health. These activities are de-
> rived from knowledge and skills from the pool of both profes-
> sional and lay experience. They are undertaken by lay people
> on their own behalf, either separately or in participative col-
> laboration with professionals.

Healing, on the other hand, is a more personal concept. As such, it is expressed
and defined in many ways. In considering healing, it is useful to remember
that the words *healing, whole,* and *holy* are derived from the same Greek word,
holos, or hale. This suggests that healing is a spiritual process that attends to the
wholeness of the person. Integration and wholeness are concepts that appear
in many definitions of healing. The following list outlines some definitions of
healing in nursing:

> **AHNA:** "A lifelong journey into wholeness, seeking harmony and
> balance in one's own life and in family, community, and global rela-
> tions. Healing involves those physical, mental, social, and spiritual
> processes of recovery, repair, renewal, and transformation that increase
> wholeness and often (though not invariably) order and coherence.
> Healing is an emergent process of the whole system bringing together
> aspects of one's self and the body-mind-emotion-spirit-environment
> at deeper levels of inner knowing, leading toward integration and bal-
> ance, with each aspect having equal importance and value. Healing
> can lead to more complex levels of personal understanding and mean-
> ing, and may be synchronous but not synonymous with curing." (2007,
> pp. 67–68)

- **Quinn:** "The emergence of right relationship at one or more levels of the bodymindspirit" (1997, p. 1).

- **Dossey, Luck, Schaub, & Keegan:** "A process of understanding and integrating the many aspects of self, leading to a deep connection with inner wisdom and an experience of balance and wholeness" (2013, p. 161).

- **Zahourek:** "Both a process and result; defined by the individual as perception of shift or meaningful change. The central concept in holistic nursing research" (2013, p. 776).

- **McElligott:** "A positive, subjective, unpredictable process involving transformation to a new sense of wholeness, spiritual transcendence, and reinterpretation of life" (2013, p. 827).

- **Cowling:** "The realization, knowledge, and appreciation of the inherent wholeness in life that elucidates prospects of clarified understanding and opportunities for action" (2000, p. 32).

There are hundreds of other well-thought-out definitions of healing. Indeed, there are likely as many different ideas about healing as there are people in this world.

The concepts of self-care and self-healing are closely intertwined and often used interchangeably. Self-care relates to health promotion and disease prevention. Self-healing—while it may encompass those aspects—also often involves a broader spiritual and transcendent component related to integration and wholeness. Although at some level it is useful to distinguish between the two, for our purposes, we will use the terms together.

Getting Started on a Plan of Self-Care and Self-Healing

Caring for ourselves is a lifelong process that involves willingness and commitment to grow and the ability to be honest with ourselves about our life circumstances. To look at life honestly, we must be able to perceive reality with clarity. Achieving clarity is a gradual process aided by introspection, reflection, and mindfulness. *Mindfulness,* which means being fully present to what is happening in our lives, fosters growth, understanding, and insight.

Following are steps you can take to develop your own plan of self-care and self-healing:

- **Be mindful and set aside time for introspection and reflection:** Making time in our day for periods of introspection and reflection is important. This may involve scheduling a 10-minute morning or evening walk, setting aside time in the evening for a relaxing bath, or creating a special time and place for a regular meditative practice and/or journaling. This is a time when we relax and allow ourselves to get in touch with our thoughts and feelings and our inner wisdom and knowingness.

    Being mindful involves staying fully present and being aware of our thoughts and feelings as we move through the day. Mindfulness is an important practice that deepens our relationship with ourselves and life and helps us to perceive reality with more clarity. Being fully present means giving full attention to what we are doing and feeling. Most often, our attention is scattered in many different directions, and we are thinking about many different things. We are mindful when we are focused on the here and now, giving full attention to the person we are with or what we are doing. This is opposed to multitasking, which involves doing several things at once and not being fully focused on anything.

ஜ **Identify areas for change:** In developing a plan of self-care, it is important for us to become aware of the patterns in our lives. What is it that we wish to focus on? Where do we want to start? What is it that we want to bring into our lives? What aspect of ourselves have we neglected? Examining the various aspects of our life and allowing ourselves time for reflection is an important step in our journey toward health and healing.

Questions for Self-Exploration and Awareness

Take some time each day to reflect on an aspect of your life. Here are some questions to help you explore various aspects of your life:

ஜ **Physical:** Is my diet optimal? Does my intake consist mainly of whole and natural foods? Do I receive optimal sleep and rest daily? Do I engage in beneficial movement and exercise daily? Do my breathing patterns promote well-being?

ஜ **Mental:** Do I have a problem-solving orientation toward life rather than a victim mentality? Do I usually have a positive attitude and positive thoughts toward work and colleagues? Do I have a sense of humor? Do I possess self-awareness? Am I objective about my strengths, limitations, and possibilities? Am I able to perceive reality with clarity?

ஜ **Emotional:** Do I love and accept myself and others? Am I able to give and receive love from myself and others? Am I able to express my own truth? Am I able to have deep feelings of identification, sympathy, and affection for others?

ஜ **Social/relational:** Do I engage in relationships that are wholesome and loving? Do I engage in relationships that promote growth in myself and others? Am I able to set healthy boundaries with others? Do I engage in work that is meaningful?

ஜ **Spiritual/energetic:** Am I able to connect with God/higher self/universe/ spirit? Do I engage in meditation/prayer/introspective practices regularly? Do I know and understand love as the essence of self? Do I have a deep respect for all?

Take your time in addressing each of these questions. Remember, this is a lifelong process of deep inner inquiry and growth. As you go through these questions, note when you respond with a powerful "no." These are the areas that need your attention. Focus on one area at a time. Create some short-term and long-term goals for each of the areas that you want to improve. Remember to treat yourself with compassion, love, and kindness!

©L. Thornton 2008, p.34, 2011, p.44.

🌿 **Set achievable goals and identify specific activities to achieve goals:** Find one or two areas that you want to change. Create a goal for each area that is realistic and achievable and then identify specific actions that will help you achieve that goal. It is important to write down your goal along with specific actions to achieve that goal. For instance, you may identify that you need to get more sleep at night.

Goal: Get 8 ½ hours sleep each night.

Specific Actions: Get children in bed by 8:00 p.m.; soak in tub from 8:10 to 8:20; be in bed by 8:30.

🌿 **Set intention and visualize results:** Setting an intention sets into motion what will happen in our lives. Take time to sit down and actually write down your intention: "My intention is to care for myself by getting at least 8 ½ hours of sleep each night." Then visualize what you will feel like and look like after accomplishing that. Imagine yourself feeling well-rested, getting up with lots of energy, and feeling optimistic and excited about the upcoming day.

🌿 **Journal or log activities:** Record how you have done each day in meeting your goals. This can be a simple tally sheet. Alternatively, you may choose to start a journal. Journaling is a wonderful way to keep track of your progress, and it also allows you to keep track of your feelings, the day's events, and your reactions and responses to all that happened. Journaling is a useful way to get in touch with some of the deeper patterns in your life, and it helps you track your progress.

- **Find a friend or support partner:** Identifying someone with whom to share the goal of creating a healthier and more wholesome life can be of invaluable assistance. Making a commitment to meet weekly or call each other daily is a good way to positively reinforce each other.

- **Be kind and compassionate toward yourself:** The process of taking care of ourselves is ongoing. It is a process that must be entered into with gentleness and an open heart toward ourselves. Many times, old patterns of making certain everything is perfect, or negative self-talk such as "This isn't going to work," "Why are you wasting so much time on yourself?" and so forth will resurface and cause setbacks. This is to be expected. When setbacks occur, simply observe them and reorient yourself toward your course of self-care and self-healing.

Summary

Self-compassion is a necessary component in caring for and healing ourselves. The three components of self compassion are self-kindness versus self-judgment, a sense of common humanity versus isolation, and mindfulness versus over-identification. These components combine to create a self-compassionate frame of mind. If we cannot feel compassion toward ourselves, we cannot care well for ourselves, nor can we care well for others. When we have closed our hearts to ourselves, we have closed ourselves to the very essence of our existence.

Mindfulness practices are important in developing a self-compassionate attitude. The practice of engaging your observer is particularly useful in dealing with emotionally charged situations and difficult social encounters. The loving-kindness meditation is another practice that is useful in cultivating love for ourselves and all human beings.

Self-compassion is linked to less anxiety, less depression, and is strongly associated with emotional intelligence and wisdom. Self-compassion is linked to greater emotional resilience and psychological well-being. Self-compassionate people are happier, have better emotional coping skills, and feel more connected to others.

Self-care and self-healing practices help us live a more balanced life and facilitate greater health, harmony, and productivity in our lives. The healthier and more balanced we are, the more effective we'll be in helping and caring for others.

The concepts of self-care and self-healing are closely related and often used interchangeably. Self-care relates to health promotion and disease prevention. Self-healing, while it may encompass those aspects, often involves a broader spiritual and transcendent component related to integration and wholeness. Some of the practices associated with self-care and self-healing include reflection, introspection, mindfulness, nutrition, exercise, massage, yoga, prayer, meditation, imagery, visualization, breathing techniques, subtle energy healing, reflexology, and acupressure.

Some of the processes involved in a self-care program include the following:

- Being mindful and setting aside time for introspection and reflection
- Identifying areas for change
- Setting achievable goals and identifying specific activities to achieve goals
- Setting intention and visualizing results
- Journaling or logging activities
- Finding a friend or support partner
- Being kind and compassionate toward yourself

References

American Holistic Nurses Association. (n.d.). Self-care practices. Retrieved from http://www. ahna.org/Membership/MemberAdvantage/Selfcare/tabid/1184/Default.aspx

American Holistic Nurses Association. (2007). *Holistic nursing: Scope and standards of care.* Silver Springs, MD: American Holistic Nurses Association & American Nurses Association.

Brach, T. (2004). *Radical acceptance: Embracing your life with the heart of a Buddha.* New York, NY: Bantam Books.

Briggs, A. (2010). The definition of self-healing. Retrieved from http://www.livestrong.com/ article/209890-the-definition-of-self-healing/

Cowling, W. R. (2000). Healing as appreciating wholeness. *Advances in Nursing Science, 22*(3), 16–32.

Dossey, M., Luck, S., Schaub, B. G., & Keegan, L. (2013). Self-Assessments. In B. Dossey & L. Keegan (Eds.), *Holistic nursing: A hand-book for practice* (6th ed.) (pp.161–187). Sudbury, MA: Jones & Bartlett.

Germer, C. (2013). Mindful self-compassion. Retrieved from www.mindfulselfcompassion.org

Kornfield, J. (1993). *A path with heart.* New York, NY: Bantam Books.

McElligott, D. (2013). The nurse as an instrument of healing. In B. Dossey & L. Keegan (Eds.), *Holistic nursing: A hand-book for practice* (6th ed.) (pp. 827–842). Sudbury, MA: Jones & Bartlett.

Neff, K. D. (2003). The development and validation of a scale to measure self-compassion. *Self and Identity, 2,* 223–250.

Neff, K. D., Hseih, Y., & Dcjitthirat, K. (2005). Self-compassion, achievement goals, and coping with academic failure. *Self and Identity, 4,* 263–287.

Neff, K. D., Kirkpatrick, K., & Rude, S. S. (2007). Self-compassion and its link to adaptive psychological functioning. *Journal of Research in Personality, 41,* 139–154.

Neff, K. D., Pisitsungkagarn, K., & Hseih, Y. (2008). Self-compassion and self-construal in the United States, Thailand, and Taiwan. *Journal of Cross-Cultural Psychology, 39,* 267–285.

Neff, K. D. (2009). Self-Compassion. In M.R. Leary & R.H. Hoyle (Eds.), *Handbook of Individual Differences in Social Behavior* (pp. 561–573). New York, NY: Guilford Press.

Neff, K. D., & McGeehee, P. (2010). Self-compassion and psychological resilience among adolescents and young adults. *Self and Identity, 9,* 225–240.

Oreg, S. (2003). Resistance to change: Developing an individual differences measure. *Journal of Applied Psychology, 88*(4), 680–93.

Quinn, J. F. (1997). Healing: A model for an integrative health care system. *Advanced Practice Nursing Quarterly, 3*(1), 1–7.

Thornton, L. (2008). Transcending differences; a holistic approach. *Imprint, 55*(5), 46–48.

Thornton, L. (2011). Self-Compassion: A prescription for well-being. *Imprint, 58*(2), 42–45.

Thornton, L. (2013). A prescription for well-being: Treating yourself right through self-care and self-compassion. *Imprint, 60*(2), 32-37.

World Health Organization. (1984). Health education in self-care: Possibilities and limitations. Health Education Services, Geneva, Switzerland. Retrieved from http://apps.who.int/iris/handle/10665/70092

Zahourek, R. (2013). Holistic nursing research: Challenges and opportunities. In B. Dossey & L. Keegan (Eds.), *Holistic nursing: A hand-book for practice* (6th ed.) (pp. 775–796). Sudbury, MA: Jones & Bartlett.

7

Self-Care and Self-Healing Practices

"Every man is the builder of a temple called his body."

–Henry David Thoreau

Chapter 1, "Shifting Toward a Paradigm of Healing and Wellness," mentioned how a large percentage of chronic disease and illness can be prevented by lifestyle changes. Eating a balanced diet consisting of whole foods, exercising regularly, and not smoking are lifestyle changes that, if implemented, could reduce the incidence of chronic disease dramatically. The World Health Organization (2005) has estimated that if the major risk factors for chronic disease were eliminated, at least 80% of all heart disease, stroke, and type 2 diabetes would be prevented, as would more than 40% of cancer cases.

Norm Shealy, MD, one of the founders of the American Holistic Medical Association, has been an advocate for a healthy lifestyle his entire career. Dr. Shealy, a neurosurgeon, developed the transcutaneous electrical nerve stimulation (TENS) unit, which has been widely used for the past several decades in physical therapy and rehabilitation clinics for nerve-related pain conditions. He quit the practice of conventional medicine and established clinics for pain and depression using primarily natural supplements, TENS units, acupuncture, and body-mind-spirit interventions. During the course of his practice, Dr. Shealy has cared for more than 35,000 clients and achieved an 85% success rate in treating patients with depression and pain, largely without the use of antidepressants or analgesics. Dr. Shealy has spent a lifetime researching technology, natural supplements, mind-body-spirit interventions, and developing programs and schools that foster wellness and heal the whole person. As outlined in the upcoming sidebar, his suggestions for creating wellness in our lives involve a healthy lifestyle, a positive attitude, and the use of natural supplements.

Essentials for a Healthy Life by Norm Shealy, MD, PhD

Health is by far the most important goal for everyone. Despite this obvious statement, 97% of Americans do not have the four essentials:

- **No smoking:** Roughly 75% of adults do follow this essential.

- **BMI (body mass index) of 18 to 24:** Less than one third of Americans meet this goal.

- **Eat minimum of five servings of fruits/vegetables daily:** Perhaps 10% of Americans meet this recommendation.

- **Exercise 30 minutes at least 5 days a week:** Approximately 10% of Americans meet this goal.

Without these four habits, little else is important. For instance, for those who smoke, there is no antidote as powerful as the poison they are taking! For those overweight and obese, there is no magic supplement that can replace proper nutrition and exercise to adjust body mass index. There are no pills that can replace whole, real food. No amount of time relaxing can compensate for inactivity.

Here are some additional suggestions:

- Laugh a lot. If you need an assistant, there are numerous CDs and DVDs that can help. You can even do a laughing meditation.*

- Check your homocysteine. If it is above 7.5, you need folic acid, B12, and vitamin C.

- Check your high sensitivity C-reactive protein. If it is above 1, have a thorough check for hidden infection.

- Deal with anger.*

- Check your cholesterol. If it is above 190, check my recommendations.*

- Take vitamin D3, 50,000 units, and K2, 100 mcg, at least once a week. This is the single best health enhancement beyond the basic four!

- Take a good multivitamin/mineral.

- Use magnesium lotion daily; 80% of Americans are deficient.

- Relax 20 minutes daily, *after* you do the essential exercise!

- Drink non-chlorinated/fluoridated water. Average eight glasses daily.

- If you have any significant symptoms, check yourself for gluten sensitivity.*

- Sleep 7 to 8 hours each night.

- If you drink alcohol, do so in moderation.

- Take a minimum of 100 mg of CoQ10 daily.

- Take a minimum of 3g of omega-3s daily.

- Avoid fast-food restaurants.

- Shop carefully and buy only whole, real (as opposed to processed) food.

- Be happy!

Reproduced with permission from Shealy, 2013.

*For more information, visit www.selfhealthsystems.com and access e-newsletter archives.

Exploring Stress and Burnout

In addition to adopting a healthy lifestyle, the topics of stress and stress management need to be explored. Indeed, the impact of stress on creating or contributing to illness and disease may be as significant as an unhealthy lifestyle. Polls show that half of all Americans say job stress affects their health, personal relationships, and/or ability to do their jobs. The estimated cost to businesses is more than $150 billion each year in absenteeism, lost productivity, accidents, and medical insurance. Some estimate that 60% of all absence from work is caused by stress-related disorders. The American Academy of Family Physicians has estimated that 60% of all problems brought to physicians in this country are stress related, and the problems that aren't directly caused by stress are made worse or last longer because of it (Hafen, Karren, Frandsen, & Smith, 1996, p. 243).

Neuroscientist and biologist Robert M. Sapolosky of Stanford Medical School (as cited in Hafen, Karren, Frandsen, & Smith, 2006) points out the pervasive effects of stress:

> As recently as 1900, the leading causes of death in America were tuberculosis, pneumonia, and flu. In just a few generations, we have conquered these and nearly all other infectious diseases, as well as those of poor hygiene and under nutrition. Suddenly, Americans live and die differently from any other humans in history and most other people on Earth. Instead of succumbing to childhood infection, or passing away in one night's malarial fever, we now survive long enough to witness the slow deterioration of our bodies—the steady clogging of arteries, the gradual weakening of the immune system until it finally lets the seed of a tumor take root. One of the most important medical insights of recent decades has been that these diseases of aging—and the pace at which they advance—can

be greatly affected by how we lead our lives, in particular, by how much stress we experience. (p. 242)

As shown in Table 7.1, the physiological effects of stress are all pervasive, affecting every system in the body.

Table 7.1 Some Effects of Stress on Organs and Body Systems

Brain	Stress kills significant numbers of vitally important brain cells. The hippocampus, which is centrally involved in learning and memory, is profoundly affected.
Immune system	Stress suppresses the production of lymphocytes (the white blood cells responsible for killing infection) and natural killer cells (the specialized cells that destroy foreign invaders such as viruses and cancer cells). It also increases T suppressors, decreases the level of interferon, and shrinks immune organs such as the thymus.
Adrenal glands	Under stress, these glands secrete large amounts of cortisone, which inhibits vitamin D activity, causing loss of calcium and a predisposition to osteoporosis.
Thyroid gland	Under stress, this gland secretes thyroid hormone, which increases metabolism. This can lead to insomnia, nervousness, heat intolerance, and exhaustion.
Hypothalamus	The hypothalamus releases endorphins. If stress is chronic, then endorphin supply becomes depleted and aggravates migraine headaches, backaches, and even arthritis pain.

continues

Table 7.1   Some Effects of Stress on Organs and Body Systems   *(continued)*

Sex hormones	Stress causes a decrease in sex hormones, loss of sex drive, infertility, and sexual dysfunction.
Cardiovascular system	Stress increases the heart rate; increases blood pressure; elevates serum cholesterol; causes blood vessels to constrict, predisposing people with arteriosclerosis to heart attacks; and causes the blood to thicken and coagulate more readily, predisposing to heart attack, stroke, and embolus.
Gastrointestinal system	Stress stops saliva production; halts the regular contractions of the esophagus or causes uncontrollable irregular contractions; increases the stomach's manufacture of hydrochloric acid; and slows stomach function, predisposing the body to ulceration. Stress disrupts the normal peristalsis of the entire intestinal tract, resulting in diarrhea or constipation. Eating while under stress can cause stomach bloating, nausea, abdominal discomfort, cramping, and/or diarrhea.
Liver	Stress causes an overproduction of glucose, increasing the risk of diabetes.
Pancreas	Stress may cause chronic inflammation of the pancreas and blockage of the pancreatic and bile ducts.
Senses	Under stress, all five senses become acute, but over an extended time, sight, hearing, taste, smell, and sense of touch become less efficient.

Compiled from: Hafen, Karren, Frandsen, & Smith, 1996, pp. 59–72.

Everyone has experienced or been aware of some of the effects of stress. No one who is conscious and living in this world is immune from the stressful factors that permeate our existence. The scary part is that the list of effects in Table 7.1 is only a partial list. Stress, along with every other emotion we experience, affects every cell and every part of our body.

There is a silver lining to this seemingly dismal cloud, however. The wonderful aspect of this is that we can control many of our responses to stress. Although we may not be able to control our environment or the stressors that are inherent parts of it, we can control our reaction to those stressors. There are tools and practices that we can incorporate into our lives that will help mediate the effects that normal day-to-day stressors can have on us. These will not work 100% of the time, but they are useful practices that can accompany us on our journey to a healthier and more wholesome way of being.

The Power of Thoughts and Emotions

Our thoughts are very powerful. Every thought precedes an action, and every action helps to create our reality. Our intentions are a powerful form of thought that sets into motion what we will create in our lives. We don't often think of our thoughts and emotions as being things, but recent research in psychoneuroimmunology and its allied fields, including neuroimmunomodulation, psychoneuroendocrinology, and behavioral medicine, have demonstrated that our thoughts and feelings enact changes in nearly every cell and organ system of the body (Pert, Dreher, & Ruff, 2005).

One remarkable discovery is that the hypothalamus produces chemicals that match every emotion that we are experiencing. In other words, for every emotion, a corresponding neuropeptide or neurohormone is produced. There are chemicals for anger, sadness, victimization, love—whatever we experience, there is a matching peptide. The moment we experience the emotion, peptides are produced and released into the bloodstream through the pituitary gland. Nearly every single cell in the body has receptor sites for nearly every neuropeptide that is produced. When these receptor sites receive a neuropeptide, a cascade of chemical and molecular changes occur in the cell (Hagelin, 2004). That means every time we experience an emotion, it alters nearly every cell in our body! This explains why Candice Pert refers to the cell as "the smallest unit of consciousness in the body" (Dispenza & Pert, 2004).

And there's more. The more you experience a particular emotion—for instance, anger—the more receptor sites are created on each cell for the neuropeptide that corresponds to that emotion. If you continue to react to situations with anger, those neuropeptides that correspond to anger will continue to flood your system, and more and more receptor sites that receive that particular neuropeptide will be created on the cells' membranes. Once receptor sites are formed, the cell naturally wants those sites to be filled with the corresponding neuropeptide. So, if you are angry on a daily basis, and you go a day or two without experiencing anger, then your body actually begins to crave those neuropeptides and unconsciously sets you up to experience anger. In essence, this means we can become physiologically addicted to experiencing certain emotions. If we notice certain patterns of emotional responses in our lives—for instance, feeling victimized or always feeling disappointed—we may actually have a physiological addiction to those emotional states (Dispenza & Pert, 2004).

Because neuropeptide receptors are not limited to the brain but are present in cells throughout the body, emotions may therefore be the bridge between the mind and body. Research from behavioral medicine has verified that our state of disease or health is inextricably linked to emotional experience. The neuropeptide network provides the physiological basis for observations from the time of Hippocrates to the modern age, that conscious and unconscious feelings are root factors in health and healing (Pert, Dreher, & Ruff, 2005). The Buddha, who knew nothing about neuropeptides, likewise affirms the power of our thoughts in the Dhammapada by saying:

> We are what we think.
> All that we are arises with our thoughts.
> With our thoughts we make the world.
> Speak or act with an impure mind
> And trouble will follow you
> As the wheel follows the ox that draws the cart.
> We are what we think.
> All that we are arises with our thoughts.
> With our thoughts we make the world.
> Speak or act with a pure mind
> And happiness will follow you
> As your shadow, unshakeable. (Kornfield, 1993, p. 283)

Thoughts and Practices That Heal

Stressful emotions can cause harmful effects in all parts of our body. Conversely, positive thoughts and emotions can promote healing and wellness. If we find ourselves repeatedly experiencing negative emotions such as anger, despair, or hopelessness, we can consciously employ practices that will shift those negative emotions toward positive and life-affirming feelings.

There are several very effective techniques that can be used to convert negative thoughts and emotions into positive thoughts that can promote healing. These practices can disrupt patterns of emotional and physiological addictions and create healthy ways of responding to people and situations. Some of the self-care techniques include:

- ⚘ Affirmations

- ⚘ Visualization

- ⚘ The Wholistic Hybrid of EFT and EMDR (WHEE) technique

These practices can be readily incorporated into our daily routines and can easily be taught to our patients and clients.

Affirmations

An affirmation is a positive statement that we develop and repeat to ourselves to change negative thoughts and feelings to positive thoughts and feelings. They are one of the quickest and most powerful ways to shift out of stress mode and into a more relaxed and calm state of being. Affirmations can help us form positive patterns of responding and break those negative response patterns that keep us from enjoying and appreciating life.

There are a few things to remember when developing affirmations:

- ⚘ **Always state the affirmation in a positive way:** For example, instead of saying, "I am not tired," say, "I am rested." This is because negations such as "not" often go unrecognized by the brain, so your brain might interpret the first statement as "I am tired."

- ⚘ **Repeat affirmations 20–30 times daily over a 3 to 5 week period.** It takes between 21 and 32 days of daily practice to form an unconscious thought pattern. During each repetition, practice repeating your affirmation a minimum of 10 times.

- ⚘ **Use reminders:** Remind yourself to practice by placing sticky notes with your affirmation in your bedroom, bathroom mirror, kitchen, car, or on your computer. Writing your affirmation on an index card that you keep in your pocket and use throughout the day is also effective.

Following are several examples of affirmations:

- I am valuable. I give and receive love.

- I speak my truth with ease and wisdom.

- I confront difficult situations and people with candidness and compassion.

- I am appreciated, and I appreciate others.

- I am complete just as I am. I am enough.

- I am a sacred child of God, precious beyond words.

- I am healthy and strong. My body is infused with vitality, health, and healing.

- I care for myself in healthy ways, each and every day.

- I have a positive attitude and welcome growth and change in my life and work.

- I am meeting people who are positive and supportive in my life.

- Peace and relaxation flow through me with every breath that I take.

- I handle all my experiences with wisdom, love, and ease.

- I am in harmony and peace within myself and in my relationships with others.

- I move through life with grace and ease; I have ample time and abundant energy to accomplish all that I must do.

I still remember the affirmation I used during a period in my life when I was trying to juggle work, school, and a young family. I constantly felt anxious about not being able to complete all that I needed to do during the day. I created the affirmation, "I move through life with grace and ease; I have ample time and abundant energy to accomplish all that I must do." Every time I began to feel the least bit of stress, I repeated the affirmation several times. After using this affirmation for several days, I became more relaxed and at ease. I also noticed that the stress-related symptoms I was experiencing such as indigestion, headaches, and insomnia subsided, and I felt energetic throughout the day. Take time to create an affirmation that meets your needs and that will help you achieve your goals and soul's purpose.

Visualization

Visualization is mentally creating a picture or image of what you want to achieve or enjoy in your life. It is a tool that you can use to help deal with any stress-producing situation. Whether the stress is related to managing a household; clinical performance; or relationships with family, friends, or coworkers, this is a tool that can help you mentally create and imagine healthy outcomes to life's many challenges. It is an excellent tool to help get rid of negative thoughts you hear in your head and can help you act in new ways that are life affirming.

There are four components to effective visualization:

- Defining your goal in clear detail
- Relaxing your body and calming your senses
- Seeing yourself achieving your goal in great detail, engaging all your senses so the outcome becomes a "felt experience"—physically, emotionally, mentally, and socially
- Practicing regularly (Thornton, 2006)

Example of Visualization

Suppose you continually find yourself in situations in which you are trying to please other people so much that you negate your own needs and are unable to speak your own truth.

To address this, create a clear goal of what you want to achieve. For example, in this case, you want to set boundaries with others that honor your needs and to speak your truth through honest and direct communication. Then, relax your body and calm your senses. Engage in whatever relaxation practice works best for you. See yourself achieving your goal in great detail. In your mind, picture the entire experience in a positive way. Imagine this is a dress rehearsal for what will manifest in your life.

- **Re-create experience:** See yourself interacting with a person whom you ordinarily want to please. For example, imagine he or she has just approached you, asking if you will do him or her a favor. You realize that your workload is already full, and you know that you cannot add another task to your day without feeling overloaded.

- **Visualize in great detail:** See yourself engaging with that person. Notice the clothes you are wearing and the clothes that he or she is wearing. Notice the setting and any particular scents that you smell or colors that you see. In your mind, create the situation with as much detail as you can possibly imagine.

- **Imagine the positive outcome:** Now, imagine your positive, self-affirming response. Rather than responding from a sense of obligation and wanting to please the person, you feel a sense of compassion for both you and the other. You breathe deeply and with a compassionate attitude respond, "I'm sorry, I would love to help you, but I already have a full workload and cannot add another task to my day."

- **Become aware of your feelings after your positive response:** Fully experience how good it feels to speak your truth and set boundaries that honor and respect who you are. Experience the compassion you feel for the other. Feel what it is like to respond from a place of knowingness and compassion that honors both you and the other person. Congratulate yourself and feel the joy of your successful response!

Remember: Old patterns take a while to reconstruct. You may not immediately change your response patterns or manifest what you want to create in your life, but with continued practice, your patterns will shift. Also remember that even if your behaviors do not immediately change, the positive thoughts that you are imagining in your dress rehearsals are already creating positive effects in your body and creating a healthier you.

The WHEE Technique

The WHEE technique is a combination of the eye movement desensitization and reprocessing (EMDR) method and the emotional freedom technique (EFT). These techniques are useful in overcoming emotional, psychological, and physical pain and challenges. The WHEE technique was developed by Dr. Dan Benor, MD, a holistic psychiatrist who had been using both techniques in his work with children but found that the children were having difficulty maintaining compliance with the exercises. He discovered an elegantly simple technique that combined elements of EMDR and EFT with the same positive results.

Broken down into its simplest components, the WHEE technique consists of describing the qualities of pain, assessing its intensity, identifying psychological issues that are associated with the origins and worsening of the pain, tapping alternately on points on the right and left sides of the body while "reprogramming" the body/mind with affirmations and a replacement statement, reassessing, and, if necessary, repeating this series of steps until the intensity score is 0 (Benor, 2009).

To use this technique, follow these steps:

1. Identify the feeling, sensation, emotion, or situation that is bothersome. Actually feel the sensation or situation so you get not only a description of it but also a felt experience. It is useful to ask your body what it is trying to tell you…then listen. For instance, after identifying what is troublesome and asking your body what it is trying to tell you, you might receive the following message: "My back feels tight, stiff, and painful, and feels burdened by too many obligations."

2. Assign a numerical level (on a scale of 1 to 10) to the severity of the pain/discomfort that you are feeling/experiencing.

3. Repeat to yourself, "Even though [description of what you are feeling—for example, 'My back feels tight, stiff, and painful, and feels burdened by too many obligations'], I love and accept myself wholly and completely."

4. Engage in bilateral movement while repeating the affirmation in step 3. You can do this inconspicuously while at your desk by alternately tapping each foot. A bilateral movement that is effective and comforting is the use of butterfly hugs. This involves crossing your arms in front of your chest, placing the palms of each hand on the upper part of the opposite arm, and then lightly and alternately tapping your upper arms with the palms of your hands. Other options include walking, jogging, tapping your hands on your thighs, etc.

5. Take a deep breath. With the exhalation, imagine that you are letting go of whatever is not useful to you—pain, tightness, a sense of being burdened, anger, frustration, sadness, etc.

6. Reassess your level of pain/discomfort/negative emotion. Repeat steps 1 through 5 until the pain/discomfort/emotion is diminished or completely absent.

I have found this technique to be one of the easiest and most effective methods to alleviate pain and deal with interpersonal conflicts and other emotional and psychological challenges and stressors. It is very easy to teach to students, patients, clients, and children. It is also a very quick way of acknowledging what we are experiencing, creating a positive affirmation to replace the negative feeling, and reprogramming our bodies for positive patterning.

Personal Experience with WHEE

During a board retreat, Dr. Benor and I were participating in a mini vision quest that involved a mountain hike. Dr. Benor noticed I was limping and asked if I would like to get rid of the pain I was experiencing. Several years prior to that, I tore all three of my hamstring muscles in my right leg completely from the bone while trying to windsurf. The hamstrings were reattached to my ischial tuberosity by miniscule molly bolts that became tender and painful upon exertion and caused me to limp. "That would be great," I responded to Dr. Benor, thinking to myself, "I've had this problem for years; it's ludicrous to hope it will disappear."

Dr. Benor asked me to get in touch with what my leg was trying to tell me. I could hear my leg respond, "I hurt. I feel overburdened, constricted, and tight." Dr. Benor said, "Fine. Now repeat out loud: 'Even though my leg hurts, and feels overburdened, tight, and constricted, I love and accept myself, wholly and completely.'" I felt rather silly at first, walking through the mountains repeating this affirmation out loud. (Walking, as a bilateral movement, takes the place of bilateral tapping or butterfly hugs.) After each repetition, Dr. Benor asked me to assess the pain level on a scale of 1 to 10. I was amazed. I first assessed my pain at a level 7. After repeating the phrase several times, my perceived pain level decreased to a 4, then to a 2, and, after about 20 minutes, the pain was completely gone!

One might attribute such an occurrence to a mountain high, a fluke interaction, or the intervention of some gnome in the forest. However, this pain has never recurred with the intensity that it had previously manifested. Dr. Benor taught me to listen to my body more carefully and to notice when it begins to feel uncomfortable. "That way," he said, "your body won't have to start screaming with pain to get your attention." So now, when I begin to feel my leg "whisper" that it is uncomfortable, I simply pay attention to it and repeat to myself, "Even though my leg feels uncomfortable, I love and accept myself wholly and completely." With one or two repetitions of this phrase, the discomfort is gone, and my leg feels fine.

Breathing Breaks to Reduce Tension and Stress

Common responses to stress include shallow breathing, holding your breath, and irregular breathing. These responses lead to greater tension and anxiety and further difficulty with breathing, which in turn leads to decreased awareness and clarity in thinking. It is possible to voluntarily activate the parasympathetic system by breathing in a slow and deliberate manner into and out of your belly. This type of abdominal breathing shuts down the stress response, enables you to relax, and places you in an optimal performance zone (Luskin & Pelletier, 2006).

Belly breathing is a wonderful technique to incorporate throughout your day. It is also a very useful technique to teach your patients who are experiencing stress and anxiety. Try this simple exercise for abdominal breathing:

1. Put your hand just under your navel.

2. Breathe deeply into the base of your lungs and expand your lower abdomen as you inhale so that you feel your hand rising as you breathe in and falling as you breathe out.

3. As you inhale count very slowly to four.

4. As you exhale, count very slowly from four back to one.

5. Repeat until you feel relaxed and calm.

There are a variety of breathing techniques that you can use to help shut down the stress response and enable you to relax in challenging situations. Take a few minutes to try each of them and determine which one feels best to you. These techniques can be practiced quickly and in any setting to elicit the relaxation response. Here are a few examples (Benson & Stuart, 1992):

  ✎ Take a deep breath and hold it for several seconds. Then, as you very slowly let your breath out, repeat a word, phrase, or prayer—for example, "Peace," "I am relaxed and at ease," "I am present to the here and now," etc.

  ✎ Put your right hand just under your navel. Focus on breathing down into your stomach, not breathing up into your chest. Your hand should rise as you breathe in and fall as you breathe out. As you inhale, say, "Ten." Exhale. With the next inhalation, say "Nine," then breathe out. Do this until you reach zero.

  ✎ Breathe in through your nose and then breathe out through your mouth. Do this 10 times. Notice how cool the air feels as you inhale in contrast to how warm it feels as you exhale.

Subtle Energy Practices That Heal

There are a variety of subtle energy practices that can be incorporated into a plan of self-care. As mentioned, subtle energy therapies have been shown to be useful in reducing stress, pain, and anxiety; accelerating healing; and promoting a greater sense of well-being. As we begin to view ourselves as fields of energy, incorporating subtle energy practices becomes foundational to self-care.

Just as our thoughts and emotions have been shown to affect our physiology and biology, our thoughts and emotions also affect the functioning of the energy centers in our body, called *chakras*. Kunz and Krieger (2004) talk about the importance of positive emotions in balancing and harmonizing the energy systems of the body:

> One way to develop the chakras so they will evenly work together is trying to be as harmonious, or integrated, in your behaviors as possible. If you get constantly upset and your

emotions are out of balance, you may function adequately for some time, but you will not experience harmony in the chakra system as a whole. It is we, ourselves, who can produce this harmony or integration. Nobody else can do it for us. It is like exercising a muscle; you, yourself, must support the coordination of the chakra system by your actions. (p. 154)

There are numerous practices and modalities that balance, modulate, and strengthen the subtle energy systems of our bodies. Some of these practices include therapeutic touch, healing touch, Reiki, Jyorei, qigong, Jin Shin Jyutsu, Pranic healing, acupressure, reflexology, and meditation, to name a few. Incorporating subtle energy practices in your daily routine can restore health and prevent illness. To become proficient in the use and application of any subtle energy modality, considerable time and practice with reputable and accomplished healers and programs is necessary.

Some subtle energy practices can be easily learned and immediately incorporated into a plan of self-care. These practices can help you become acquainted with your "subtle energy body." The following is a sampling of techniques to introduce you to subtle energy practices. These techniques are useful for your personal health and can be taught to patients and clients to provide relaxation and a sense of well-being and to alleviate a variety of symptoms.

Jin Shin Jyutsu

Jin Shin Jyutsu is an ancient healing art, similar to acupressure and acupuncture, that uses gentle pressure of the hands to stimulate the energy flow within the body, restoring balance and harmony. Releasing accumulated tension and stress enables the body to heal itself (Jin Shin Jyutsu, 2013). Two self-care Jin Shin Jyutsu practices are particularly easy and useful: harmonizing the main central vertical flow and harmonizing finger holds.

Harmonizing the Main Central Vertical Flow

In Jin Shin Jyutsu, the main central vertical flow is considered the source of our life energy. This pathway flows down the center of the front of the body and up the back of the body. Harmonizing the main central vertical flow is a self-care practice that balances and stimulates the flow of energy throughout the body (see Figure 7.1). This practice can be easily accomplished while lying down as well as while sitting in a chair. This self-care practice is useful in balancing the energies in your body before going to sleep at night or upon waking.

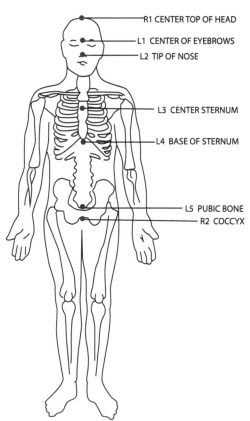

Figure 7.1 Harmonizing the main central vertical flow (Segal, 1976).

To harmonize the main central vertical flow, follow these steps (reprinted with permission from Jin Shin Jyutsu, Inc.):

1. Place the fingers of the right hand on the top of the head (where they will remain until step 6). Place the fingers of the left hand on your forehead between your eyebrows. Hold for 2 to 5 minutes or until the pulses you feel at your fingertips synchronize with each other.

2. Move the left fingertips to the tip of the nose. Hold them there for 2 to 5 minutes or until the pulses synchronize.

3. Move the left fingertips to your sternum at the center of your chest. Stay there for 2 to 5 minutes or until the pulses synchronize.

4. Move your left fingers to the base of your sternum (at the center of where your ribs start, above the stomach). Hold them there for 2 to 5 minutes or until the pulses synchronize.

5. Move your fingers to the top of your pubic bone (above the genitals, at the center). Hold them there for 2 to 5 minutes or until the pulses synchronize.

6. Keep your left fingertips in place and move your right fingertips to cover your coccyx (tailbone). Hold them there for 2 to 5 minutes or until the pulses you feel at your fingertips synchronize with each other.

Note

The right hand remains on the top of the head while the left hand moves down the body until the final step.

Harmonizing Finger Holds

The practice known as the harmonizing finger holds method promotes relaxation and a sense of calm and peacefulness. The phrase "Get rid of worry FAST" is used to describe this practice, with FAST being an acronym for the emotions of fear, anger, sadness, and "try to's" (pretenses). Each finger corresponds to an energy meridian that is related to a specific emotion. Holding the fingers helps balance the energies associated with the various emotions (see Figure 7.2).

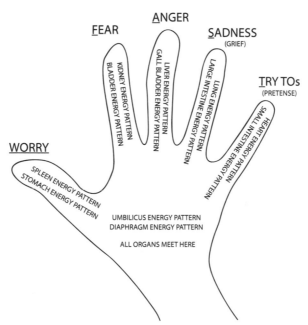

Figure 7.2   Harmonizing finger holds (Segal, 1976).

To harmonize the finger holds, follow these steps (reprinted with permission from Jin Shin Jyutsu, Inc.):

1. Sit or recline in a comfortable position and close your eyes.

2. Take a couple of soft, deep breaths in through your nose and out through your mouth.

3. Breathe naturally and focus your attention on your breathing.

4. Gently wrap the fingers of your right hand around your left thumb.

5. Hold this position until you feel a gentle, soothing pulsation or for a minimum of 1 minute.

6. One by one, repeat steps 4 and 5 on each of your fingers.

7. If time permits, repeat all the steps on the other hand.

Alternative approaches include beginning with either hand (the choice is yours) and, if you prefer, shifting back and forth between hands (e.g., thumb to thumb, index finger to index finger, etc.).

Reflexology

Reflexology is an ancient healing art based on the premise that there are zones and reflex areas in the feet and hands that correspond to all body parts and systems. These areas can be lined up with the foot by imagining that the human body is superimposed on the foot. This is called the *theory of reiteration,* meaning that the feet are actually a mirror image of the body (see Figure 7.3 and Figure 7.4). The physical act of applying specific pressures using the thumb, finger, and hand techniques results in stress reduction, which promotes positive physiological changes in the body (American Reflexology Certification Board, 2013).

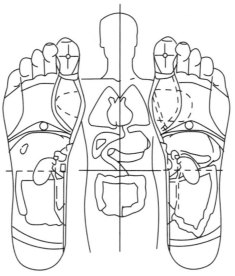

Figure 7.3   A mini map of the whole body.

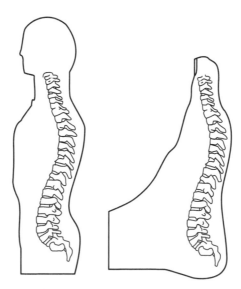

Figure 7.4   The inside curves of the foot correspond to the curves
of the spine.

Research studies conducted around the world, including in the United States, have validated the effectiveness of reflexology on a wide variety of conditions. Chronic conditions seem to respond especially well to reflexology. In China, where reflexology is accepted by the central government as a means of preventing and curing diseases and preserving health, more than 300 research studies have shown reflexology provided some improvement to 95% of the more than 18,000 cases covering 64 illnesses studied (American Reflexology Certification Board, 2013). In Japan and Denmark, reflexology has been incorporated into the employee health programs of several large corporations and demonstrated considerable savings by decreasing the amount of paid sick leave benefits (Ericksen & Levin, 1995).

Reflexology can be used as a self-care practice. Reflexology charts of the feet and hands (see Figure 7.5 and Figure 7.6) show the points that correspond to various organs and parts of the body. For instance, if you are experiencing tightness or pain in your back, simply look at the charts, identify those areas that correspond to the area of your back that is problematic, and massage either your hands or feet in those areas. If you are feeling low on energy, massaging the area corresponding to your adrenal glands often provides an added boost of energy. Generally, points on your feet or hands that are extremely sensitive indicate areas of energy congestion. Massaging those areas helps to increase circulation and energy flow and to improve your overall sense of well-being.

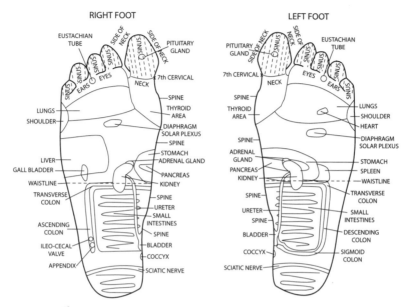

Figure 7.5 A reflexology chart of the feet (Segal, 1976).

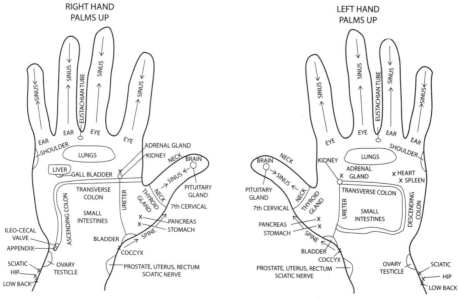

Figure 7.6 A reflexology chart of the hand (Segal, 1976).

Acupressure

The role of acupressure has been paramount in traditional Chinese medicine (TCM) for more than 2,000 years. Acupressure is essentially a method of sending a signal to the body to turn on its own self-healing or regulatory mechanisms. Normally, *qi* (vital energy) circulates through natural pathways in the body called *meridians*. Blockage of this flow, or an imbalance in *yin* and *yang*, can cause illness and pain. Acupressure helps to correct functional imbalances and restore flow, thus returning the body to a more natural state of well-being (UCLA Center for East-West Medicine, 2012). You can use acupressure to treat a variety of conditions and symptoms. It is a wonderful way to get in touch with your subtle energy body and restore and harmonize your energy flow.

As shown in Figure 7.7, there are five essential acupressure points (Source: UCLA Center for East-West Medicine, 2012. Reproduced with permission from the UCLA Center for East-West Medicine):

- **Large intestine 4 (LI 4):** This point is located at the highest spot of the muscle when the thumb and the index fingers are brought close together. This point is good for stress, headaches, toothaches, facial pain, and neck pain. However, as a word of caution, it can induce labor and must never be used during pregnancy.

- **Pericardium 6 (P 6):** Turn your hand over so that your palm is facing up to the ceiling. Locate the crease where your wrist and hand connect. This is the point located about three fingers breadth above that crease and is midway between the two large bones in your arm. This point can help provide relief for nausea, anxiety, carpal tunnel syndrome, upset stomach, motion sickness, and headaches, and is even used for regulation of heart palpitations.

✍ **Liver 3 (Liv 3):** You need to take off your shoe to find this point. It is located about two finger widths above the place where the skin of your big toe and next toe joins. This is an excellent area to stimulate for stress, low back pain, high blood pressure, limb pain, insomnia, and emotional upset.

✍ **Stomach 36 (St 36):** Find this point by measuring four finger widths down from the bottom of your knee cap. Then, cut across toward the outside of your leg. You'll find it about one finger breadth from the outer boundary of your shin bone. If you are in the right place, a muscle should pop out as you move your foot up and down. You can find this point useful for fatigue and depression as well as knee pain and gastrointestinal discomfort. Asians frequently stimulate this point for health promotion and longevity.

✍ **Spleen 6 (Sp 6):** Find the bony mound on the inside of your leg close to your ankle. From the top of this bump, measure four finger widths up your leg and push at the area just slightly behind the leg bone. This point can be very helpful for many urological and pelvic disorders as well as fatigue and insomnia. Avoid during pregnancy.

To stimulate the acupressure points, press firmly with a finger in a rotary movement or an up-and-down movement for several minutes at a time (UCLA Center for East-West Medicine, 2012).

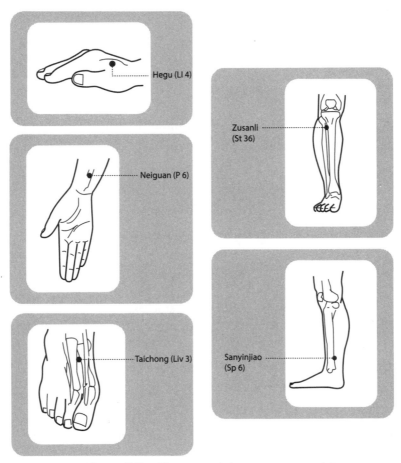

Figure 7.7   Five essential acupressure points.

Summary

A large percentage of chronic disease and illness can be prevented by lifestyle changes. Not smoking, eating a balanced diet consisting of whole foods, and exercising regularly are lifestyle changes that, if implemented, could dramatically reduce the incidence of chronic disease.

The impact that stress has on creating or contributing to illness and disease may be as significant as an unhealthy lifestyle. The American Academy of Family physicians has estimated that 60% of all problems brought to physicians in the United States are stress related, and the problems that aren't directly caused by stress are made worse or last longer because of it (Hafen, Karren, Frandsen, & Smith, 1996, p. 243). Programs that care for the whole person must include components of stress management.

Stress affects every system of the body. It has adverse effects on the brain, immune system, cardiovascular system, gastrointestinal system, reproductive system, liver, adrenal glands, pancreas, and all of our senses. Recent advances in the field of psychoneuroimmunology have demonstrated that stressful thoughts and feelings create adverse physiological effects in almost every cell of our bodies. Also, our cells can become physiologically addicted to experiencing certain emotions. That means unhealthy emotional patterns may be deeply embedded in the physiology of our bodies.

The use of self-care and self-healing practices can help reprogram our thoughts and feelings, reestablish healthy ways of being, and create healthier bodies. Using techniques such as affirmations, visualization, and the WHEE technique are ways that we can create healthier patterns in our life and mitigate the negative effects of stress.

The use of conscious breathing practices is an easy and effective way to shut down the stress response and enable us to relax during challenging times. When we are stressed, our sympathetic system engages, and we usually respond with shallow breathing, holding our breath, or irregular breathing. Using conscious breathing practices such as belly breathing, or other slow and deliberate breathing techniques, voluntarily activates the parasympathetic system and enables us to relax.

There are a variety of body-based and subtle energy practices that are very useful in balancing and unblocking the flow of energy and helping us relax. Subtle energy and body-based practices that can be incorporated into a self-care practice include therapeutic touch, healing touch, Reiki, Jyorei, qigong, Jin Shin Jyutsu, acupressure, and reflexology, to name a few.

An important aspect of developing a self-care program is getting in touch with your body, mind, heart, and soul. It is critical to deeply listen to those parts that you have shut off or neglected. When you use affirmations and visualization, you are taking time to relax and imagine what you want to create in your life. To do this, you must get in touch with how you are presently feeling. The WHEE technique engages you in a process of asking your body what it is trying to tell you. You must listen and hear your body's message. When we engage in deep abdominal breathing, we are moving our consciousness back into our body and quieting our system so that our perspective can broaden and we can respond from a place of clarity. When we incorporate the practices of harmonizing the main central vertical flow and the harmonizing finger holds, we are paying attention to the flow and pulsations of energy and learning to get in touch with our subtle energy body. Incorporating the practice of reflexology and acupressure helps us become aware of the meridians in our body and of how the different points on our body are connected to various organs, systems, and other parts of our body. Caring for ourselves is an ongoing process that involves a variety of approaches and practices that will change throughout the course of our life.

References

American Reflexology Certification Board. (n.d.). American Reflexology Certification Board: Welcome to ARCB. Retrieved from http://arcb.net/cms

Benor, D. (2009). *Seven minutes to natural pain release.* Bellmawr, NJ: Wholistic Healing Publications.

Benson, H., & Stuart, E. (1992). *The wellness book: The comprehensive guide to maintaining health and treating stress related disorders.* Seacaucus, NJ: Carol Publishing Group.

Dispenza, J., & Pert, C. (2004). Interviewed in Chasse, B. & Arntz, W. (Producer). (2004). *What the bleep do we know* [Motion picture]. USA: Captured Light Industries. Retrieved from www.whatthebleep.com

Eriksen, L., & Levin, S. (1995). *A closeup view on company reflexology* (Committee Report): Danish Reflexologists Association.

Hafen, B. Q., Karren, K. J., Frandsen, K. J., & Smith, L. N. (1996). *Mind/body health: The effects of attitudes, emotions, and relationships.* Needham Heights, MA: Allyn & Bacon.

Hagelin, J. (2004). Interviewed in Chasse, B. & Arntz, W. (Producer). (2004). *What the bleep do we know* [Motion picture]. USA: Captured Light Industries. Retrieved from www.whatthebleep.com

Jin Shin Jyutsu. (2013). Jin Shin Jyutsu: The art of getting to know (help) myself. Retrieved from http://jsjinc.net/index.php

Kornfield, J. (1993). *A path with heart.* New York, NY: Bantam Books.

Kunz, D., & Krieger, D. (2004). The spiritual dimension of therapeutic touch. Rochester, VT: Bear & Company.

Luskin, F., & Pelletier, K. (2006). *Stress free for good.* New York, NY: Harper Collins.

Pert, C., Dreher, H., & Ruff, M. (2005). The psychosomatic network: Foundations of mind-body medicine. In M. Schlitz, T. Amorock, & M. Micozzi (Eds.), *Consciousness & healing: Integral approaches to mind-body medicine* (pp. 61–78). St. Louis, MO: Elsevier Churchill Livingstone.

Segal, M. (1976). *Reflexology.* Los Angeles, CA: Wilshire Book Company.

Shealy, N. (2009). Essentials for a healthy life. Retrieved from https://normshealy.com/news-letter/read.asp?news=218#.UXK1sMrfyyA

Thornton, L. (2006). Certificate program in transformational healthcare leadership: CDModule1: Stress hardiness. Creating a healing environment. Fresno, CA.

UCLA Center for East-West Medicine (2012). *Five essential acupressure points.* Santa Monica, CA: UCLA Health System.

World Health Organization. (2005). *Preventing chronic diseases: A vital investment.* Geneva, Switzerland: World Health Organization. Retrieved from http://www.who.int/chp/chronic_disease_report/full_report.pdf

8

Optimal Health and Wellness

*"May your life be an awakening and may you
see each choice as the dawning of a new you."*

–Anonymous

Note

The majority of this chapter was contributed by C.M. Thornton, JD, MA).

In the model of whole-person caring, optimal health and wellness occurs when we have integrated our highest potential into every aspect of our lives. This is a lifelong journey that involves valuing who we are, appreciating the preciousness of our existence, and treating ourselves with loving-kindness in all that we do. It is about living consciously: being aware of what we eat, how we care for our bodies, who we bring into our lives, the quality of our relationships, and the meaning and usefulness of our work.

Manifesting Optimal Wellness

Optimal wellness involves every aspect of ourselves. Within the WPC model, the spiritual/energetic essence provides the foundation for optimal wellness. It is at this foundational level that unconditional love arises and a person's meaning in life and respect for all beings originates. As the spiritual/energetic essence (our highest potential) is integrated into the various aspects of life (e.g., physical, mental, emotional, social/relational), patterns of optimal wellness manifest.

For instance, when our highest potential is integrated into the mental aspect of our being, certain characteristics will manifest in our lives. We will have the ability to perceive reality with more clarity. This means that many of the filters that have shrouded our vision will gradually disappear and we will see life as it is, rather than how we have been conditioned to see it. Another manifestation in the mental realm is that we will become more self-aware. We will be more objective about our strengths, limitations, and possibilities. Many of the dramas that have played over and over in our lives will gradually disappear as we begin to give less attention to the negative patterns that we have created.

In the emotional realm, the integration of our highest potential will manifest in many different ways. For example, we will have a greater acceptance and appreciation for ourselves. Cultivating a compassionate attitude will positively affect how we care for ourselves in every way. This compassion will spill into our relationships with others. We will find that we can begin to love and accept others without judgment and criticism. We will also find that we begin to have a deeper appreciation and sense of gratitude for the basic pleasures of life.

When our highest potential is integrated into our social/relational dimension, we will find that the relationships in which we engage become more wholesome and loving. We will bring relationships into our lives that promote growth in ourselves and others. Gradually, relationships that are negative and not rooted in love and kindness will move to the periphery of our lives.

When our highest potential is integrated into our spiritual life, we will feel a connection with all that is. We may perceive this as a connection to God, our higher self, the universe, or spirit. We will find that we regularly engage in meditation and prayer and adopt a reflective approach to life. We begin to see all of life as sacred and appreciate each person as a precious gift. Table 8.1 lists manifestations of optimal wellness.

Table 8.1   Manifestations of Optimal Wellness

Physical	Optimal dietary intake
	Optimal elimination
	Optimal rest and sleep
	Optimal movement/exercise
	Optimal breathing
Mental	Ability to perceive reality with clarity
	Self-awareness: objective about strengths, limitations, and possibilities
	Problem-solving orientation toward life: not a victim or pawn mentality
	High degree of imagination and creativity
	Positive attitude and thoughts
	Sense of humor
Emotional	Acceptance of self, others, and nature
	Ability to give and receive love from self and others
	Ability to express one's own truth
	Ability to have deep feelings of identification, sympathy, and affection for others
	Appreciation and gratefulness for basic pleasures of life

continues

Table 8.1   Manifestations of Optimal Wellness *(continued)*

Social/relational	Engaging in relationships that are wholesome and loving
	Engaging in relationships that promote growth of self and others
	Engaging in work that is meaningful
	Engaging in work that utilizes strengths and aptitudes
Spiritual/energetic	Connecting with God/higher self/universe/spirit
	Regularly engaging in meditation/prayer/introspective practices
	Knowing and understanding love as an essence of self
	Deriving meaning and purpose in life
	Cultivating a deep respect for all

Source: Gold & Thornton, 2000, p. E–1.

From the perspective of the whole person, when we change one aspect of our lives, the positive effects spill into other areas. So even though we may talk about the mental, emotional, and physical aspects, from a whole-person perspective, everything is interrelated and inseparable. Practices that can help create healthy and wholesome patterns in the emotional, mental, and social/relational dimensions of our lives were discussed in Chapter 7, "Self-Care and Self-Healing Practices." The remainder of this chapter focuses on creating optimal physical wellness, with special emphasis on nutrition and exercise.

Optimal Physical Wellness

So how do we achieve optimal physical health? The journey to optimal physical health is a dynamic and highly individualized process. We can look to science to provide viable approaches, but no universal recipe exists. It can be tempting to adopt a ready-made plan with predetermined meals and workouts, but the best plan is personalized, through a process of trial and error, to meet individual needs. The information presented here reflects established scientific knowledge to help discriminate between valid approaches and unfounded gimmicks. These broad guidelines for healthy living (i.e., eating a nutritious diet, regularly moving your body, and getting adequate sleep) provide a foundation from which to personalize and refine an individualized approach to optimal health.

Realizing optimal health is a lifelong journey that requires constant course adjustments. The diet and exercise routine that worked for you at age 25 probably will not serve you well at age 60. Changes in your environment, the availability of new products, and new research findings may inspire a modification to your routines. Realizing optimal physical health requires experimentation, an open mind, and periodic reflection as to whether your adopted practices need modification. There are endless permutations of what optimal physical health looks and feels like; amending your vision of optimal health as you grow and evolve is a fun and rewarding part of the process. This chapter provides foundational principles that you can draw on as you develop, revise, and modify your routines for optimal health.

Optimal Nutrition

The foods we choose have a cumulative effect on our health, quality of life, and risk for chronic disease. Four of the ten leading causes of death in the United States—heart disease, cancer, stroke, and diabetes—are associated with unhealthy diets. Moreover, estimates suggest that approximately one third of all cancer and heart disease is caused in part by poor diet, inactivity, and alcohol use, with the costs of diet-related chronic disease reaching $200 billion annually in medical care and lost productivity (Nestle, 2007).

Many people complain that making nutrition choices is difficult due to the flood of confusing, ever-changing nutrition advice. Yet fundamental nutrition guidelines have changed little in the past half century. For example, in 1959, Ancel Keys, a physician-researcher, and his wife, Margaret, published guidelines for prevention of heart disease—and they still hold true today.

 ## The Keyses' 1959 Dietary Guidelines

- Do not get fat. If you are fat, reduce.
- Restrict saturated fats, the fats in beef, pork, lamb, sausages, margarine, and solid shortenings, and fats in dairy products.
- Prefer vegetable oils to solid fats, but keep total fats under 30% of your diet calories.
- Favor fresh vegetables, fruits, and nonfat milk products.
- Avoid heavy use of salt and refined sugar.
- Good diets do not depend on drugs and fancy preparations.
- Get plenty of exercise and outdoor recreation.
- Be sensible about cigarettes, alcohol, excitement, busy-ness, and strain.
- See your doctor regularly, and do not worry.

Source: Keys & Keys, 1959.

Confusion arises because most nutrition advice comes from the media and the food industry. The media tends to focus on recent research "breakthroughs," which lack reliability because findings have yet to be repeated and confirmed to establish scientific consensus. News stories tend to focus on a single nutrient and rarely discuss findings in a broader dietary context. The tried-and-true dietary guidelines (e.g., "Eat more vegetables") are simply not newsworthy (Nestle, 2007). Advertising messages from the food industry are similarly unhelpful, as they market single nutrients to sell a specific product but have no incentive to promote the foundational principles of a healthy diet.

Unfortunately, no government agency has a budget to promote dietary guidelines in a fashion that can compete with the food industry's advertising. In 2000, Phillip Morris (Kraft Foods, Inc., Jell-O desserts, etc.) spent more than $2 billion advertising its packaged food products, while PepsiCo spent more than $1 billion (Nestle, 2007). In 1999, McDonald's spent $627 million, Burger King $403 million, and Taco Bell $206 million in direct media advertising (Nestle, 2007). Making healthy choices in spite of ubiquitous and often misleading advertisements can be challenging, but reliable sources of health and nutrition information, such as those listed here, are a good place to start.

Government Health Agencies

- **MedlinePlus (www.medlineplus.gov):** Sponsored by the National Library of Medicine and National Institutes of Health, this source provides reliable information on a variety of health topics, including an excellent review of the safety and efficacy of many supplements and herbs.

- **PubMed (www.ncbi.nlm.nih.gov/pubmed):** To help you do your own research, the National Library of Medicine's PubMed.gov website offers free access to scientific research papers. The database is easy to use and offers instructions for beginners.

- **Healthfinder (www.healthfinder.gov):** This site offers reliable health information sponsored by the U.S. Department of Health and Human Services.

- **Nutrition.gov (www.nutrition.gov):** This website, sponsored by the National Agricultural Library and the Food and Nutrition Information Center, provides information to help improve dietary patterns, including links to USDA's MyPlate and Dietary Guidelines for Americans.

✐ Professional Health Organizations

- **American College of Sports Medicine (www.acsm.org):** This professional organization is committed to using scientific research to maintain and enhance physical performance, fitness, health, and quality of life.

- **American Dietetic Association (www.eatright.org):** This professional organization is dedicated to promoting health through nutrition.

Despite the confounding deluge of news and advertisements, broad dietary guidelines have remained constant: Eat a primarily plant-based diet, low in saturated fats, sodium, and added sugars. Research has shown that populations with the longest lifespan, including several Asian and Mediterranean populations, tend to eat relatively low-calorie diets that are high in vitamins, minerals, fibers, and other plant compounds (phytochemicals) and rely less on foods from animal sources (Nestle, 2007).

The dietary guidelines for Americans echo these principles, setting forth two overarching concepts:

- ✐ Maintain calorie balance over time to achieve and sustain a healthy weight.

- ✐ Focus on consuming nutrient-dense foods and beverages.

The guidelines recognize that

> Americans currently consume too much sodium and too many calories from solid fats, added sugars, and refined grains.… A healthy eating pattern limits intake of sodium, solid fats, added sugars, and refined grains and emphasizes

nutrient-dense foods and beverages—vegetables, fruits, whole grains, fat-free or low-fat milk and milk products, seafood, lean meats and poultry, eggs, beans and peas, and nuts and seeds. (U.S. Department of Agriculture [USDA] and U.S. Department of Health and Human Services [USDHHS], 2010, p. ix)

Calorie Control and Optimal Weight

Maintaining optimal weight can be challenging in America's "obesogenic" society, which promotes overconsumption, unhealthy food choices, and inactivity (Dunford & Doyle, 2012). We drive to get fast food, have pizza delivered to our home, and even stand on escalators while going *down*. Due to our culture of excess consumption and inactivity, a whopping 64% of women and 72% of men are overweight or obese, with about one third of adults being obese (USDA & USDHHS, 2010). To beat the odds and maintain optimal health, it is necessary to control caloric intake to match energy expenditure. To estimate energy intake and expenditure, use online calculators from Shape Up America!, a nonprofit organization committed to the promotion of physical activity and healthy eating (www.shapeup.org/resources/tools_index.html).

How can we get all the nutrients we need without consuming too many calories? The key is choosing nutrient-dense foods—foods that contain a relatively high concentration of nutrients for the calories they contain. For example, ice cream and nonfat milk both provide calcium, but milk has greater nutrient density because it provides more calcium per calorie. Fruits and vegetables are nutrient dense because they are low in calories but contain a lot of vitamins and minerals. In contrast, sugar and alcohol have low nutrient density because they contain empty calories, without providing vitamins, minerals, or protein. (Mazzeo & Mangili, 2013). A good rule is to choose whole, unprocessed foods, as processing often strips foods of nutrients or fiber and adds calories in the form of fat or sugar.

Techniques such as recording dietary intake, using smaller plates, and eating only in designated places in the house can also help reduce caloric intake. Conscious eating practices are also effective at teaching nutritious eating habits. Following are examples of conscious eating habits:

- Eat in a calm atmosphere. Create traditions such as lighting candles and using cloth napkins to create a warm and loving atmosphere. No TV, radio, or reading books.

- Take a moment to express gratitude for the food. This can be done out loud or in silence. Create a special blessing that honors the food and everyone involved in its production. Create an intention of what the energy of this food will be used for, such as "May this food provide the energy that will sustain and heal my life and those around me."

- Never eat when you are upset.

- Sit down and relax. Always sit down to eat and refrain from eating on the run. Take a couple of deep abdominal breaths and allow your belly to relax before eating.

- Eat slowly and consciously. After each bite, chew your food slowly and consciously, and refrain from taking another bite until you have completely chewed and swallowed the previous one.

- Eat only when you feel hungry.

- Avoid ice-cold food and drink. According to Ayurvedic medicine, cold drinks decrease digestive fires and can cause indigestion. Sip warm water with your meals. Adding lemon to warm water helps aid digestion. Don't drink too much liquid, as it dilutes the enzymes that break down your food.

- Eat with full attention and gusto. Enjoy!

  ✎ Leave one third to one quarter of your stomach empty to aid digestion.

  ✎ Wait until one meal is digested before eating the next (e.g, intervals of 2 to 4 hours for light meals or 4 to 6 hours for full meals).

  ✎ Sit quietly after your meals.

Making Wise Nutrition Choices

Our abundant food supply provides many options, so it is important to learn how to choose wisely. The healthiest diets are primarily plant-based, focusing on unprocessed foods such as fruits, vegetables, whole grains, and legumes, while limiting consumption of refined carbohydrates, processed foods with added sugar, saturated fat, trans fat, and sodium.

Carbohydrates

Carbohydrates are an essential part of a healthy diet, providing a wealth of needed vitamins, minerals, fiber, and phytochemicals. However, not all carbohydrates are created equal. Complex carbohydrates such as fruits, vegetables, and whole grains should form the foundation of our diets. Most Americans eat too many refined grains, especially those that have been processed to add sugar, fat, and sodium. In fact, the top source of calories for Americans is grain-based desserts—cookies, cake, pastries, etc. (Mazzeo & Mangili, 2013). Refined carbohydrates are digested rapidly, causing blood-glucose levels to quickly rise and fall, leaving us hungry and wanting to eat more. In contrast, complex carbohydrates are digested more slowly, which means glucose enters the bloodstream more gradually, keeping us full for longer.

Added Sugars and Their Pseudonyms

Check food labels for these hidden added sugars: dextrose, maltose, sucrose, glucose, lactose, corn syrup, high-fructose corn syrup, malt syrup, evaporated cane juice, cane sugar, fruit juice concentrate, molasses, honey, agave, and brown sugar (Bushman, 2011).

Do carbohydrates make us fat? It has been suggested that rising obesity rates may be related to increased carbohydrate consumption. However, blaming carbohydrates is a mistake. Many cultures consume high-carbohydrate diets, yet they maintain low rates of obesity. Rising obesity is the result of an increase in overall caloric consumption combined with decreased physical activity. Any type of food is fattening if you eat more calories than you expend. Carbohydrates consist of the nutrient-rich plant-foods that provide the basis for a healthy diet (Sizer & Whitney, 2012).

Do low-carbohydrate diets work? Research has shown that low-carbohydrate diets can help people lose weight quickly in the short term but are no more effective than any other reduced-calorie diet in the long term. People on low-carbohydrate diets tend to consume fewer calories because they eliminate a broad category of food from their diet; however, the long-term success of weight loss relates to the maintenance of restricted calorie intake, not the proportion of carbohydrate and protein consumed (Sizer & Whitney, 2012). High-protein, low-carbohydrate diets also raise several health concerns. Protein-rich foods contain more saturated fat and cholesterol, which are associated with chronic disease. Moreover, omitting whole grains, fruits, vegetables, and milk also eliminates important nutrients, fiber, and phytochemicals with proven health benefits. Finally, high-protein diets may place undue stress on the kidneys and may harm bone health due to increased excretion of calcium (Dunford & Doyle, 2012).

Fat

Fat is another macronutrient that receives undeserved criticism. Like carbohydrates, fat is an essential part of a healthy diet—as long as you choose wisely and consume it with moderation. As a general rule, "good" fats come from plant and fish sources, while "bad" fats come from animal sources or processed foods. Approximately 20–35% of your calories should come from fat, with less than 10% coming from saturated fats. Intake of trans-fatty acid should be kept to a minimum. Table 8.2 outlines various types of fats, their sources, and their effects on blood lipids.

Table 8.2   Types of Fats

Type of Fatty Acid	Source	Effects on Blood Lipids
Saturated	Animal sources (meat, cheese, egg yolk, butter) and tropical oils (coconut oil and palm oil)	Raises total cholesterol and raises LDL ("lousy") cholesterol
Trans	Margarines and commercially baked goods (cookies, pies, desserts)	Raises total cholesterol and raises LDL ("lousy") cholesterol
Monounsaturated	Olive oil, canola oil, peanut oil, and avocado	Lowers total cholesterol, lowers LDL ("lousy") cholesterol, may raise HDL ("healthy") cholesterol
Polyunsaturated	Vegetable oils (corn oil, soybean oil, sesame oil, safflower oil, sunflower oil, flaxseed oil) and fish	Lowers total cholesterol, lowers LDL ("lousy") cholesterol, may raise HDL ("healthy") cholesterol

Remember, whether the fats are saturated or unsaturated, all fats supply 9 calories/gram—more than twice the number of calories in protein or carbohydrates. For weight management, what matters is the total number of calories eaten, but eating a low-fat diet is a good way to stay within your caloric limits. Fats in our diet can be visible (oils, butter, fat trimmed from a steak) or invisible (marbling of meat; fats blended into sauces of mixed dishes; fat ground into lunch meats and hamburger; fats in nuts, avocados, or olives; fats in baked and fried foods). It is important to read the label. For example, ground chicken and ground turkey often have skin, heart, and liver ground into the meat, making them high in fat (Duyff, 2012; Dunford & Doyle, 2012).

Interpreting Food Labels

Fat-free: Less than ½ gram of fat per serving

Low-fat: 3 grams or less of fat per serving

Reduced fat: At least 25% less fat per serving compared to traditional food

Protein

Most Americans easily meet their protein needs. A wide variety of foods contain protein, including the usual suspects (meat, poultry, fish, and dairy products), as well as numerous vegetarian options (legumes, beans, lentils, vegetables, and grains) (Dunford & Doyle, 2012). Proteins from animal sources can be high in saturated fat, so choose lean meats and low-fat dairy products. When choosing meat, a cut with "loin" or "round" in the name generally contains less fat (Duyff, 2012).

As you make improvements to your diet, remember that optimal nutrition doesn't require perfection. Our bodies remember what we do *most* of the time, so practice self-compassion, go at your own pace, and enjoy your journey to optimal health. Table 8.3 contains a summary of healthy eating guidelines.

Table 8.3   Summary: Healthy Eating Guidelines

Carbohydrates	Choose fiber-rich fruits, vegetables, and whole grains.
	Limit sugar, processed foods with added sugar, and refined carbohydrates (white bread, white rice).
Fats	Choose unsaturated fats, found in plant and fish sources.
	Limit saturated fat, trans fat, and cholesterol, found in animal sources and processed foods.
Protein and dairy	Choose lean meat and low-fat/nonfat dairy products.
	Limit red meat, butter, and cream (high in saturated fat).

Supplements

Most experts agree that it is better to obtain nutrients from whole foods, not pills and powders. Foods contain non-nutrients such as phytochemicals, which have disease-fighting properties but cannot be extracted and replicated in supplement form. Foods also contain fiber and water, nutrients essential to digestive and overall health. That being said, the supplement industry has now made available a wide array of herbs and botanicals. Many supplements reflect traditional remedies that have been used by other cultures to promote health for thousands of years. This section provides information to help you make smart choices when it comes to buying a supplement.

Supplements include a wide variety of products including vitamins, minerals, botanicals, and herbs. Vitamins and minerals have been studied for years and produce well-documented health effects (Nestle, 2007). Most vitamins and minerals have established standards (dietary reference intakes) for amounts needed by humans, and many have established tolerable upper intake levels, which set the maximum daily dosage. If you choose to buy a multivitamin as insurance against a potential nutrient deficiency, choose a product that does not contain nutrients in amounts exceeding 150% of the recommended dietary allowance (RDA) and take it only every other day to avoid toxicity (Sizer & Whitney, 2012).

In contrast to vitamins and minerals, research on herbal and botanical supplements is in its infancy, and most herbal and botanical supplements have not undergone scientific study needed to define active ingredients, determine safety, or evaluate efficacy to produce claimed health outcomes. Standardization of herbal supplements presents a unique challenge because the dosage of active ingredients can vary depending on the plant species and location, the part of the plant used, the age at harvest, the preparation technique (for example, cutting produces different results than mashing), the processing, and the method for extraction (Dunford & Doyle, 2012). Thus, an effective traditional herbal remedy may have a different composition (and effect on health) when it undergoes Western processing and packaging.

Unlike most European nations, which regulate herbals and botanicals as medications, the United States deregulated supplements with the passage of the 1994 Dietary Supplement Health and Education Act (DSHEA) (Dunford & Doyle, 2012). Pursuant to DSHEA, manufacturers have no duty to prove that a supplement is safe or effective before selling it to the public. Instead, the FDA has the burden to prove that the supplement is unsafe and must undergo a protracted and costly process, including filing and winning a lawsuit, before the product is withdrawn (Nestle, 2007).

In 2007, the Food and Drug Administration mandated quality standards (good manufacturing practices) intended to ensure that supplements contain the ingredients listed on the label and do not contain contaminants (Dunford & Doyle, 2012). The FDA is now taking action to enforce the standards but faces a great challenge given the sheer number of supplements on the market. In 2009, the FDA reported that more than 70 weight loss supplements were tainted with prescription drugs not listed on the label (Dunford & Doyle,

2012). In 2010, the Government Accountability Office reported findings of toxic contaminants such as lead, mercury, cadmium, and arsenic in herbal dietary supplements (Dunford & Doyle, 2012).

Ultimately, the responsibility lies with the consumer to make educated choices. The first step is determining which nutrients, if any, are lacking in one's diet. Research shows that most people take supplements that they do not need and do not take supplements containing nutrients missing in their diet (Sizer & Whitney, 2012). Free online dietary analysis programs, such as the USDA's SuperTracker (https://www.supertracker.usda.gov/) or Sparkpeople (www.sparkpeople.com), can be used to track dietary intake and identify potential deficiencies or toxicities.

Before purchasing a supplement, check whether the manufacturer has obtained certification from an independent laboratory such as the National Science Foundation (www.nsf.org) or United States Pharmacopeia (www.usp.org). These companies test and certify that the supplement contains the ingredients listed on the label. (Note, however, that certification does not confirm the safety or effectiveness of the product.) Finally, refrain from buying the newest "magic pill" or trendy supplement. If a product sounds too good to be true, it probably is. By following these guidelines and making educated choices, you can feel confident in your use of supplements.

Optimal Physical Fitness

Engaging in regular physical activity is one of the most effective and accessible means of improving and maintaining both physical and mental health. Many leading chronic diseases (heart disease, diabetes, hypertension) can be described as *hypokinetic*—diseases that result from inadequate levels of physical activity. Along with increasing longevity and decreasing risk of disease, maintaining physical fitness offers immediate benefits such as increasing self-confidence, boosting mood, increasing energy, and improving quality of sleep.

Emerging research also shows that physical activity affects mental functioning by creating the ideal "chemical soup" in the brain to facilitate learning, decrease stress and anxiety, alleviate depression, and treat dementia (Ratey & Hagerman, 2008). While most drugs used for mental health target only one type of neurotransmitter (e.g., Prozac targets serotonin; Ritalin targets dopamine), physical activity positively affects all of the brain's neurotransmitters and hormones, creating an optimal and natural chemical balance (Ratey & Hagerman, 2008). If you are looking for a miracle cure, physical activity is just that. This section provides an overview of how to implement a safe, effective, and well-balanced fitness program. It covers the major components of physical fitness, including aerobic fitness, muscular fitness, and flexibility (Thompson, 2010).

Exercise the Blues Away

In the landmark Standard Medical Intervention and Long-term Exercise (SMILE) study, researchers compared the effects of taking the SSRI sertraline (Zoloft) with exercise for treating depression. The 156 participants were divided into three groups treated with Zoloft, exercise, or both. At the end of 16 weeks, the results showed that exercise was just as effective as Zoloft at reducing depression. Moreover, the 10-month follow-up showed that participants in the exercise group had lower rates of relapse into depression as compared to the Zoloft group (Blumenthal, Smith, & Hoffman, 2012).

Aerobic Training

When we challenge our body with aerobic training, we stimulate physiological and metabolic adaptations that improve our ability to take in oxygen, deliver oxygen and nutrients to working tissue, and generate energy (Kenney, Wilmore & Costill, 2012). These adaptations not only decrease risk for chronic disease, but also they increase our daily quality of life by increasing our available energy to accomplish tasks throughout the day.

There are many physiological benefits of aerobic training. For example, aerobic training (Kenney, Wilmore & Costill, 2012, pp. 248–270):

- Improves circulation, which facilitates delivery of oxygen and nutrients throughout the body

- Increases the effectiveness of the heart muscle's capability to pump blood

- Increases stroke volume, the amount of blood ejected by the heart during contraction

- Decreases the resting heart rate as the heart becomes more efficient and can pump more blood per contraction

- Increases the total blood volume, which improves circulation

- Promotes growth of new capillaries to facilitate better blood flow

- Decreases blood pressure in individuals with hypertension or borderline hypertension

- Increases myoglobin, which carries and delivers oxygen to working tissue

- Increases mitochondria, the organelle responsible for converting oxygen and nutrients into usable energy

Aerobic training includes any rhythmic exercise engaging large muscle groups (e.g., walking, jogging, cycling, swimming, or cross-country skiing). The American College of Sports Medicine (ACSM), the leading professional organization in exercise science, recommends engaging in a *minimum* of 150 minutes of aerobic exercise per week (30 minutes per day, 5 days per week) to maintain cardiopulmonary health. For greater health and fitness benefits, and to prevent weight gain, 250–300 minutes per week (50–60 minutes per day, 5 days per week) is required. If the goal is weight loss, some individuals may need to progress to as much as 60–90 minutes per day, 5 to 7 days per week (Thompson, 2010).

Each exercise session should begin with a slow, low-intensity, sport-specific, progressive warm-up for 5 to 10 minutes. The goal of the warm-up is to increase heart rate, core temperature (create a mild sweat response), joint range of motion, and blood flow to working muscles. A proper warm-up will reduce risk of musculoskeletal injury, cardiac incident, and post-exercise soreness.

For health and fitness purposes, the ACSM recommends a combination of both moderate intensity and vigorous intensity exercise (Bushman, 2011). Equipped with both fast-twitch and slow-twitch muscle fibers, the human body is designed to engage in exercise of varying intensity levels (e.g., walking, jogging, and sprinting). As exercise intensity increases, we increase the overload on our body, which responds with greater physiological adaptation. In addition to facilitating more significant increases in cardiovascular and muscular fitness, high-intensity exercise has been shown to decrease body fat and increase post-exercise metabolism to a greater extent than low-intensity exercise (Yoshioka et. al., 2001).

The Talk Test

The talk test provides a simple and reliable method to measure exercise intensity (Bushman, 2011):

- **Low intensity:** You can talk and sing without labored breathing.
- **Moderate intensity:** You can comfortably talk, but not sing.
- **High intensity:** You cannot say more than a few words without gasping for breath.

Each exercise session should end with a cool-down, consisting of 5 to 10 minutes of low- to moderate-intensity activity. The cool-down allows the heart rate and blood pressure to recover, prevents blood from pooling in extremities, and allows blood to circulate and remove any accumulated metabolic wastes (e.g., lactic acid) (Thompson, 2010).

Strength Training

Strength training is an integral part of a balanced fitness program, providing a host of health benefits. Strength training improves body composition by increasing lean muscle mass, thereby increasing the resting metabolic rate (the amount of calories you burn at rest). Theoretically, gaining two pounds of muscle will increase your resting metabolic rate by approximately 21 calories per day (Bushman, 2011). Strength training also improves bone density. When your muscles pull on the bone during a strength exercise, your body responds by building more bone cells to manage the increased demand. Other benefits of strength training include the following:

- Improved balance

- Decreased risk of injury

- Toned appearance

- Counteraction of age-related muscular atrophy

As with aerobic training, the benefits of strength training are both immediate, increasing day-to-day capabilities, and long-term, decreasing risk of injury and chronic diseases such as heart disease and osteoporosis (Bushman, 2011).

A variety of strength-training equipment can be used to improve muscular fitness—for example, weight machines, free weights, body weight, balls, and bands (Thompson, 2010). The key is finding the most convenient and comfortable mode of training to increase adherence to the training program. When starting out, take care not to do too much too soon. Overreaching leads to fatigue, decreased motivation, and increased risk of injury. Also be sure to receive instruction on proper technique to avoid injury and ensure effective training (Thompson, 2010).

The ACSM recommends training each major muscle group (chest, shoulders, upper and lower back, abdomen, hips, and legs) 2 to 3 days per week, allowing at least 48 hours before working the same muscle group (Thompson, 2010). Train each muscle group for 2 to 4 sets, with 8 to 12 repetitions per set, and take 2 to 3 minutes of rest between sets. For a very deconditioned individual or an older adult, use slightly lighter weights and decrease the volume to one or more sets of 10 to 15 repetitions (Thompson, 2010).

When selecting a weight, choose one that can you can lift for only 10 repetitions (on the first set) before becoming fatigued. If you can complete more than 10 repetitions, you need a heavier weight. If you can complete fewer than 8 repetitions, select a lighter weight. When you can complete 15 repetitions on the first set, it is time to progress to the next weight. Remember, it is necessary to overload the muscles to see an increase in muscular fitness (Bushman, 2011).

Flexibility Training

Flexibility is generally the most overlooked and underappreciated component of fitness, yet it is necessary to maintain a high quality of life. Flexibility allows us to move our bodies freely and fluidly—to bend down and tie our shoes, to look over our shoulder to back up the car, or to reach up to get something on a high shelf.

Stretching is most effective when muscles are warm and can be performed after the warm-up or at the end of the workout. Spend at least 10 minutes stretching, addressing each major body part (Bushman, 2011). Stretch each muscle to the point of mild tension, holding for 15 to 30 seconds, with 4 repetitions per stretch (Thompson, 2010). Like other aspects of fitness, flexibility will improve with a consistent effort. Table 8.4 contains a summary of exercise recommendations for healthy adults (Thompson, 2008).

Table 8.4   Summary: Exercise Recommendations for Healthy Adults

Aerobic exercise	150 minutes per week (30 minutes per day, 5 days per week) minimum to maintain cardiopulmonary health.
	250–300 minutes per week (50–60 minutes per day, 5 days per week) to prevent weight gain and obtain greater health and fitness benefits.
	For weight loss, some individuals may need to progress to as much as 60–90 minutes per day, 5 to 7 days per week.
Strength training	Perform a full-body workout 2 to 3 days per week.
	Train each major muscle group: chest, shoulders, back, abdomen, hips, and legs.
	Do 2 to 4 sets, with 8 to 12 repetitions per set.
Flexibility	Stretch when muscles are warm, after a warm-up or at the end of a workout.
	Stretch for at least 10 minutes, 2 to 3 times per week.
	Hold each stretch for 15–30 seconds.

Steps to Fitness Success

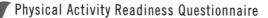Physical Activity Readiness Questionnaire

1. Has your doctor ever said that you have a heart condition and that you should only do physical activity recommended by a doctor?
2. Do you feel pain in your chest when you do physical activity?
3. In the past month, have you had chest pain when you were not doing physical activity?
4. Do you lose your balance because of dizziness, or do you ever lose consciousness?
5. Do you have a bone or joint problem (for example, back, knee, or hip) that could be made worse by a change in your physical activity?
6. Is your doctor currently prescribing drugs for your blood pressure or a heart condition?
7. Do you know of any other reason why you should not do physical activity?

If you answered yes to one or more of these questions, see your doctor before you start becoming much more physically active or before you have a fitness appraisal.

When goal setting, select goals that are specific, realistic, and within your control. For example, the goal "Improve cardiovascular health" is not specific or measurable. A better goal might be "Run a mile in under 9 minutes." Similarly, setting a goal to "Lose 10 pounds in a week" is probably not realistic nor within your control. Instead of focusing on the weight-loss outcome, set a goal to guide the process: "I will walk 5 times this week, 45 minutes per session, at a brisk pace." This goal is specific, action-oriented, and within your control.

Following are some tips for making exercise a positive experience (Anshel, 2006):

- Choose a type of aerobic exercise you enjoy.

- Make an exercise calendar and schedule exercise sessions just as you would any other important appointment.

- Set achievable goals.

- Gradually increase duration and intensity of exercise to prevent injury.

- Ensure social support.

- Find a convenient exercise environment that feels safe and comfortable.

- Record baseline fitness measures so you can see improvement and feel a sense of achievement.

- Go at your own pace and avoid feelings of competitiveness or the need to meet others' standards.

- Develop pre-exercise rituals to make exercise a regular part of your day.

- Create a plan for dealing with and overcoming setbacks such as missing a workout, illness, injury, loss of social support, lack of progress, not meeting goals, stressful life events, etc.

- Exercise to your favorite music.

- Add variety to your workout and incorporate fun recreational activities.

Achieving optimal health means more than having acceptable health markers and avoiding chronic illnesses. Optimal health is a state of being that facilitates the achievement of higher goals and purposes. With optimal health and wellness, we can actively pursue our passions, spend meaningful time with our families, develop healthy relationships, and engage in meaningful work. Optimal health provides us with strength and confidence to overcome obstacles, grow, and evolve. Whether we are pursuing our dreams or enjoying an everyday experience, optimal health and wellness allow us to reach our highest potential.

Summary

In the model of whole-person caring, optimal health and wellness occur when we have integrated our highest potential into the various aspects of our lives. This is a lifelong journey that involves valuing who we are, appreciating the preciousness of our existence, and treating ourselves with loving-kindness in all that we do. As the spiritual/energetic essence (our highest potential) is integrated into the various aspects of life (e.g., physical, mental, emotional, social/relational, spiritual), patterns of optimal wellness manifest. Optimal wellness might manifest in the different aspects of our lives as follows:

- **Physical:** Optimal diet and exercise
- **Mental:** Ability to perceive reality with more clarity
- **Emotional:** A greater acceptance of self and others
- **Social/relational:** Engaging in relationships that are wholesome and loving
- **Spiritual:** A closer connection to God/spirit.

The fundamental guidelines for optimal nutrition have not changed over the years: Eat a plant-based diet low in saturated fats, sodium, and added sugars. Research has shown that populations with the longest lifespan, including several Asian and Mediterranean populations, tend to eat relatively low-calorie diets that are high in vitamins, minerals, fibers, and other plant compounds (phytochemicals) and rely less on foods from animal sources. Confusion arises because most nutrition advice comes from the media and the food industry.

Due to our culture of excessive consumption and inactivity, 64% of American women and 72% of American men are overweight or obese, with about one third of adults being obese. Yet we can get all the nutrients we need without overconsuming calories by choosing nutrient-dense foods—foods that contain a relatively high concentration of nutrients for the calories they contain. For example, fruits and vegetables are nutrient dense because they are low in calories but contain a lot of vitamins and minerals. In contrast, sugar and alcohol have low nutrient density because they contain empty calories without providing vitamins, minerals, or protein.

Most experts agree that it is better to obtain nutrients from whole foods, not pills and powders. Food contains non-nutrients such as phytochemicals, which have disease-fighting properties but cannot be extracted and replicated in supplement form. Research shows that most people take supplements that they do not need and do not take supplements containing nutrients missing in their diet. Online dietary analysis programs, such as Sparkpeople or the USDA's SuperTracker, can be used to track dietary intake and identify potential deficiencies or toxicities. Refrain from buying the newest "magic pill" or trendy supplement. If a product sounds too good to be true, it probably is.

Engaging in regular physical activity is one of the most effective and accessible means of improving and maintaining both physical and mental health. A combination of aerobic exercise (swimming, running, cycling, brisk walking), strength training (lifting weights, using bands), and flexibility exercise (stretching, yoga, Pilates) should be combined for maximum benefit. Optimal health and wellness is a state of being that facilitates the achievement of higher goals and purposes and allows us to reach our highest potential.

References

Anshel, M. H. (2006). *Applied exercise psychology: A practitioner's guide to improving client health and fitness.* New York, NY: Springer Publishers.

Blumenthal, J., Smith, P. & Hoffman, B. (2012). Is exercise a viable treatment for depression? *ACSM's Health & Fitness Journal, 16*(4), 14–21.

Bushman, B. (2011). *ACSM's complete guide to fitness and health.* Champaign, IL: Human Kinetics.

Dunford, M., & Doyle, J. A. (2012). *Nutrition for sport and exercise.* Belmont, CA: Wadsworth.

Duyff, R. L. (2012). *American Dietetic Association complete food and nutrition guide* (4th ed.). Hoboken, NJ: John Wiley & Sons, Inc.

Gold, J., & Thornton, L. (2000). *Creating a healing culture: Whole-person caring.* Gold & Thornton Publishing.

Keys A., & Keys M. (1959). *Eat well and stay well.* New York, NY: Doubleday.

Kenney, L., Wilmore, J., & Costill, D. (2012). *Physiology of Sport and Exercise* (5th ed.). Champaign, IL: Human Kinetics.

Mazzeo, K., & Mangili, L. (2013). *Fitness!* (5th ed.). Belmont, CA: Wadsworth.

Nestle, M. (2007). *Food politics: How the food industry influences nutrition and health.* Berkeley, CA: University of California Press.

Ratey, J. & Hagerman, E. (2008). *Spark: The revolutionary new science of exercise and the brain.* New York, NY: Little, Brown and Company.

Sizer, F. & Whitney, E. (2011). *Nutrition concepts and controversies* (12th ed.). Belmont, CA: Wadsworth.

Thompson, W. (2010). *ACSM's guidelines for exercise testing and prescription* (8th ed.). Philadelphia, PA: Lippincott Williams & Wilkins.

U.S. Department of Agriculture and U.S Department of Health and Human Services. (2010). Dietary Guidelines for Americans (7th ed.). Washington, DC.: U.S. Government Printing Office. Retrieved from www.dietaryguidelines.gov

Yoshioka, M., Doucet, E., St-Pierre, S., Almearas, N., Richard, D., Labrie, A., Labrie, A.,…, Tremblay, A. (2001). Impact of high-intensity exercise on energy expenditure, lipid oxidation and body fatness. *International Journal of Obesity, 25,* 332–339.

9

Therapeutic Partnering and Transformational Leadership

"True compassion only occurs among equals."

–Dalai Lama

Therapeutic partnering and transformational leadership are key concepts of the model of whole-person caring. Together, these concepts help organizations bring to life a caring and healing environment. In the model of whole-person caring, the foundation for all relationships and all leadership is based in the spiritual-energetic realm. So while therapeutic partnering and transformational leadership are different concepts, what supports and enlivens them is the same.

Therapeutic Partnering

Therapeutic means to promote health and healing. Partner is defined as one with whom we share a common mission and purpose. A healthy partnership is characterized by mutual respect, compassion, trust, and clear communication. Combining these concepts, the definition of therapeutic partnering in the WPC model is as follows:

> A relationship between people whose common mission and purpose is to promote healing and wellness and is characterized by mutual power, respect, compassion, trust, and clear communication.

In therapeutic partnering, the relationships of partners are based on healing. Mutual power means that there is equality of power, and while the knowledge bases of individuals may be different, there is no hierarchy based on education or status within the organization or community. Each member of the partnership is regarded with mutual respect, compassion, trust, and appreciation. People are brought together with a common goal and purpose to promote healing and wellness.

When we talk about therapeutic partnerships, there are two primary relationships that are of interest to us. The first is the relationship between the health care provider and the patient. The second is the relationship between health care providers and practitioners of other disciplines.

Cultivating Therapeutic Partnerships with Our Patients

What does it mean to have a relationship based in health and healing? How is that different from the traditional relationship between health care providers and their patients? What characterizes a healing relationship? Further, how is a relationship that is characterized by mutual power, respect, compassion, trust, and clear communication different from the more traditional relationship that exists between health care providers and the people they serve?

Creating a Field of Healing

In the model of whole-person caring, the person is viewed as a spiritual and sacred being. Each person is seen as a precious gift who is to be treated with the utmost kindness, dignity, respect, and love. The health care provider creates sacred space when caring for the person. The provider does this through a process of centering themselves and accessing their spiritual self, where feelings of love and compassion naturally arise. This state is referred to as being *heart centered*. Research has shown that a heart-centered state creates a coherence in the electromagnetic field with many positive emotional and physiological effects (McCraty & Reese, 2009). Basically, health care providers access the essence of their being, their spiritual dimension, when delivering care. The consciousness of the health care provider creates a field of healing. A person who receives this type of care experiences a deep level of caring and often a feeling of being healed.

Note

Sacred space and *heart centered* are terms used in holistic nursing. They are discussed in greater detail in Chapter 10, "Caring as Sacred Practice."

Another remarkable aspect of this interaction is that health care providers are actually revitalized through this encounter. The health care provider benefits from the positive effects that are generated through the field of healing just as much as the person receiving care. This is a wonderful antidote to compassion fatigue, which is so prevalent among nurses and caregivers. Health care providers can be taught the process of becoming heart centered and use it in every patient encounter. This is a practice that enriches the care that we give to our patients as well as enriches and enlivens our own lives and work.

Empowering People

In addition to creating a healing environment, therapeutic partnering fosters self-empowerment. The traditional relationship between the health care provider and the patient is not a partnership. The traditional relationship gives more power to the health care provider based on his or her education and knowledge.

In therapeutic partnering, the patient is a partner in his or her plan of care and treatment. The health care provider brings expertise in identifying and diagnosing the problem or illness and suggests a plan of care or treatment that would be appropriate. In providing holistic care, the practitioner might identify behavioral and social patterns that are contributing to an individual's health challenges and bring these patterns to the person's awareness. Whether the provider is identifying patterns or diagnosing and suggesting a plan of care, the next process involves mutually deciding on a course of action. This engages the patient in his or her own care and creates accountability for his or her health. The health care provider is not telling the patient what he or she should do, but uses his or her own expertise to make observations and suggest options to restore or promote health and healing. The patient ultimately decides what he or she will do and is in control of decisions regarding his or her own health. In the present system, people can decide what care they will or will not receive, but the underlying assumption is that the patient will comply with whatever is recommended.

Therapeutic partnering empowers patients to take control of their health, which is foundational in moving toward a system of illness prevention and health promotion. Engaging in healthy lifestyle practices is an internally motivated process. Providing people with the tools and education they need to succeed is important, but change can occur only when the person is motivated from within. Therapeutic partnerships help empower people to take control of their health and create a healing environment that promotes health and well-being. Table 9.1 outlines the differences between traditional relationships between health care providers and their patients and therapeutic relationships.

Table 9.1   Traditional Relationships Versus Therapeutic Partnerships Between Health Care Providers and Patients

Traditional Relationship	Therapeutic Partnership
The patient is viewed as a biomedical entity.	The patient is viewed as a spiritual and sacred being.
Patients' rooms and procedure and treatment rooms are places where care is given.	In addition to providing care, patients' treatment and procedure rooms are sacred spaces where healing can occur.
The provider's focus is task centered and sometimes patient centered.	The provider's focus is whole-person centered, with an awareness of body/mind/heart/spirit.
The provider does not engage in centering.	The provider is heart centered and consciously creates a field of healing.
The provider has power and authority.	The provider and the patient are partners with equal power.
The provider diagnoses, plans, and treats.	The provider assesses, informs, educates, and suggests treatment, which is implemented in collaboration with the patient.
The patient is expected to comply with the treatment or plan of care and is a passive participant in care.	The patient and provider mutually determine the plan of care, and the patient is an active participant in his or her care.
The patient depends on the provider for health care directives.	The patient is empowered to take control and is encouraged to initiate health-promoting behaviors.

Cultivating Therapeutic Partnerships with Coworkers

The health care team is composed of a variety of partnerships. In addition to the many colleagues in our own discipline, we interact with a variety of people from other departments and disciplines. Therapeutic partnering values each department and team member as equally important. A partnership recognizes that every member of the team is crucial in providing the best possible care. The patient is the focus of all care, and members of the team are unified in a common mission and purpose to promote health and healing and to deliver the highest quality of care possible. (See Figure 9.1.)

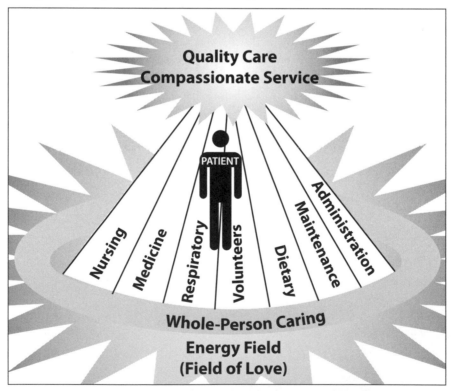

Figure 9.1   Concept of therapeutic partnerships.

The concepts in the model of whole-person caring guide us in our interactions with coworkers. Each colleague is perceived as an infinite and sacred being and deserves to be treated with respect, compassion, trust, and appreciation. Caring and healing practices are valued, and each member of the team helps create a nurturing, healthy, and healing environment. Each team member uses centering to facilitate caring and healing interactions with other team members, just as in patient interactions.

Using the concepts of the model of whole-person caring, Table 9.2 offers some ideas to reflect on to help cultivate therapeutic partnerships within your organization.

Table 9.2   Cultivating Therapeutic Partnerships with Coworkers

Whole-Person Caring Concepts	Practices and Ideas to Foster Therapeutic Partnerships
Spiritual and sacred nature of being	Be aware of how you speak and respond to each other.
	Remember that each person is a sacred being—a precious gift.
	Cultivate heart-centered communication and listening skills.
Therapeutic partnering	Treat every member of the team with respect, compassion, trust, and appreciation.
	Focus on the shared mission to promote health and healing.
	Remember: The patient is the focus of all services. It is an honor and privilege to be part of a team that provides compassionate and quality care.

continues

Table 9.2   Cultivating Therapeutic Partnerships with Coworkers *(continued)*

Whole-Person Caring Concepts	*Practices and Ideas to Foster Therapeutic Partnerships*
Self-care and healing	Encourage team members to care well for themselves.
	Develop strategies to relieve team members so each team member has adequate time for meals and breaks.
	Incorporate stress-reducing practices (e.g., WHEE technique, belly breathing, etc.) and encourage and remind team members to do likewise.
Optimal whole-person	Take your break with someone from another wellness department and walk around the organization's grounds. Incorporate deep-breathing and stretching exercises for extra energy.
	Schedule a potluck once a month and invite members of other departments to bring a healthy, low-fat dish.
Transformational leadership	Use or create unit governing councils to regularly include an agenda item that assesses the quality of relationships.
	Post the commitments to coworkers on relationship-based care or similar commitments derived from staff or other sources.

Table 9.2   Cultivating Therapeutic Partnerships with Coworkers *(continued)*

Whole-Person Caring Concepts	*Practices and Ideas to Foster Therapeutic Partnerships*
Caring as sacred practice	Teach staff the processes of centering, being a healing presence, and creating sacred space to use with patients and coworkers.
	After receiving a report, gather your team, take a couple of deep breaths together, and create a group intention, such as "Let's remember that we are here for the greater good of the patient, to promote health and healing, and to support each other in delivering the highest quality and most compassionate care possible."
	Remember that your intention sets into motion what will happen.

Therapeutic Partnerships in Integrative Health Care

The concept of therapeutic partnering is particularly useful in the integrative health care setting. Integrative health care involves combining the practice of complementary and alternative medicine (CAM) and conventional medicine.

Various models have been used in integrative medicine (IM). These models range from practitioners in private practice who offer acupuncture and energy work for their patients to freestanding institutions that offer a full complement of CAM practitioners along with conventional physicians. Many different models have evolved. Some integrative practices function under the same roof, while others use referrals to off-site practitioners.

Templeman and Robinson (2011) have identified two types of partnerships in IM models:

- **Inequitable partnerships:** In inequitable partnerships, hierarchical relationships are dominant. Medical practitioners act as the primary health care provider and CAM practitioners take on subordinate roles with a lower level of autonomy. This is the most commonly described model in the literature. Generally, the needs of the patient are not the central focus of practices that have inequitable partnerships (Templeman & Robinson, 2011). Therapeutic partnering is difficult to implement in this type of practice because the hierarchical model is antithetical to partner-based relationships.

- **Equitable partnerships:** There is a correlation between patient-focused care and equitable partnerships. Organizations that put the needs and preferences of the patient above all else tend to develop equitable partnerships. Several authors have reported that being patient focused is actually a prerequisite for an equitable partnership (Anderson, 2000; Leckridge, 2004; Peters, Chaitow, Harris, & Morrison, 2002). These partnerships adopt a more collaborative and equal power approach in decision-making, intervention, and evaluation. "This mutually empowering and supporting partnership combines the best of both CAM and conventional medicine to address the particular needs of the client, and may be particularly relevant for specific client populations such as chronic or complex health conditions, non-pharmaceutical approaches to treatment, illness prevention, and health maintenance and promotion" (Templeman & Robinson, 2011, p. 87).

Therapeutic partnering is a valuable asset for integrative health care practices that are client focused. Relationships that promote mutual power, respect, compassion, and trust, as well as clear communication between CAM practitioners and conventional practitioners, facilitate the delivery of quality care. Patients will be better served by a team that collaborates to provide the best care possible. As practitioners learn to work together, valuing and respecting each other's contributions, new and more effective ways of caring for people will evolve. When practitioners work together from a place of heart-centered communication, they create a healing environment for themselves and their clients.

As we evolve in our practices, a day will come when the labels of "CAM" and "conventional medicine" slip away and we embrace all practices that heal as healing practices. This will require working together to determine which practices are effective and which are not. It will also require that we create research methodologies that are appropriate to the study of CAM and we begin to value practice-based evidence. We must work together and replace our territorial issues with our passion to create a healthier world. Moving toward therapeutic partnerships—relationships that heal—is a step in the right direction. To do this, however, we must place the patient first!

CLEAR Communication: A Heart-Centered Approach to Communication

Experts have identified four characteristics as the foundation for healthy teams (Koloroutis, 2004):

- **Trust:** Trust encompasses both functional trust and trustworthiness. Functional trust involves such things as knowing a team member can do the job he or she was hired to do. Trustworthy people can form trusting relationships through their integrity and maturity. In the clinical setting, they exhibit competence in clinical, interpersonal, critical thinking, creative thinking, and leadership skills.

    ✤ **Mutual respect:** Mutual respect means that people are appreciated and valued because of who they are, not for their position, title, or status.

    ✤ **Consistent and visible support:** Consistent and visible support means that team members can always count on each other and will support each other in good times as well as when mistakes occur.

    ✤ **Open and honest communication:** Open and honest communication is characterized as being direct and truthful.

All these elements are crucial in relationships that foster healing. In addition, the elements of compassion and mutual power are essential for therapeutic partnerships.

In the model of whole-person caring, we use the term *CLEAR communication*. CLEAR is an acronym for the process involved in whole-person communication. It stands for Center, Listen, Empathize, Attention, and Respect. This has been a useful tool to help people remember some of the important aspects of holistic communication.

Communication: Be CLEAR

Center Yourself

    ✤ Pause for a moment.

    ✤ Breathe deeply.

    ✤ Connect with a feeling of love and compassion.

    ✤ Create a silent intention that thoughts, words, and actions will be for the greater good.

Listen Wholeheartedly

- Set aside your own thoughts, emotions, and feelings.
- Focus on the person's agenda.
- Don't judge or analyze.
- Open your heart to what is being communicated.

Empathize

- Come from a place of genuine concern.
- Ask yourself: How does this person perceive the situation? What does the world look like through this person's eyes? What is he or she feeling?
- Empathy involves an understanding that comes from sensing into the being of another.

Attention: Be Fully Present

- Be aware of what you are feeling and sensing. Stay present to yourself.
- Bring the fullness of yourself to every moment—emotionally, mentally, physically, and spiritually.

Respect

- Respect all that is.
- Respect yourself. Set boundaries if needed.
- Respect the person. Honor cultural, social, ontological, and ideological differences.
- Welcome diversity.

Source: Thornton (2006).

The purpose of the model is to remind us to access our sacred and spiritual nature in everything we do. This is not something that we can achieve 100% of the time. If we can remember even 5% or 10% of the time, we will be making great strides. The model challenges us to bring our very best, our highest nature, to all that we do.

CLEAR communication, likewise, is a reminder to engage our higher selves when we are communicating with another. Whether it is a team member or a patient, when we are centered and listening deeply, with full presence, respect, and empathy, the interaction nurtures us and the other. We have created by our very consciousness a healing presence where love and caring are palpable. This is how communication manifests in a therapeutic partnership.

Leadership in Health Care

Effective leadership is critical in the delivery of high-quality health care services. As our health care system continues to increase in complexity, the need for responsive and effective leadership will also increase. This increased need, coupled with the documented shortage of nurse leaders, makes developing and retaining health care leaders a priority. It is important, therefore, to determine which type of leadership style and focus creates the best outcomes for patients and staff.

Leadership styles can be placed in two categories based on their focus (Cummings et al., 2010, p. 364):

- Those focused on relationships, or relationally focused leadership
- Those focused on tasks, or task-focused leadership

The most common relationally focused leadership style is transformational leadership. Some common task-focused leadership styles include management by exception, laissez-faire, and transactional leadership. Each style has its own distinct characteristics. Although leaders typically have a predominant approach, they often incorporate elements from a variety of styles. Table 9.4 outlines various leadership styles and their key characteristics.

Table 9.3   Leadership Styles and Key Characteristics

Leadership Style	Characteristics
Transformational	Motivates through vision.
	Instills pride, faith, and respect, and has a gift for seeing what is important and transmitting a sense of mission.
	Focuses on meaning, purpose, values, morals, and ethics.
	Oriented toward long-term goals.
	Serves as a role model for followers.
	Encourages creativity.
	Promotes critical thinking and problem solving.
	Acts as coach and advisor.
	Keeps lines of communication open.
	Recognizes the contributions of each member.
	Encourages followers to reach goals that help both the individual and the organization.
	Challenges the status quo.
	Empowers followers to propose new and controversial ideas without fear of punishment or ridicule.
	Offers followers the opportunity to see meaning in their work and challenges them with high standards.
Transactional	Emphasizes the transaction or exchange that takes place among leaders, colleagues, and followers to accomplish the work.
	Preoccupied with power and position, politics, and perks.
	Mired in daily affairs.
	Focuses on tactical issues.
	Follows and fulfills role expectations by striving to work effectively within current systems.

continues

Table 9.3   Leadership Styles and Key Characteristics   *(continued)*

Leadership Style	Characteristics
	Supports structures and systems that reinforce the bottom line.
	Maximizes efficiency and guarantees short-term profits.
Management by exception	Practice whereby only the information that indicates a significant deviation of actual results from the budgeted or planned results is brought to the managers' attention.
	Its objective is to facilitate managers' focus on really important tactical and strategic tasks.
	Decisions that cannot be made at one level of management are passed on to the next higher level.
	Focuses on monitoring tasks and execution for any problems that might arise and correcting those problems to maintain current performance levels.
Laissez-faire	Uses a non-authoritarian leadership style.
	Laissez-faire leaders give the least possible guidance to subordinates and try to achieve control through less obvious means.
	Laissez-faire leaders believe that people excel when they are left alone to respond to their responsibilities and obligations in their own ways.
	Incorporates passive avoidance of issues, decision-making, and accountability.

Sources: Avolio, Bass, & Jung, 1999; Bass & Avolio, 1994; Covey, 1992; Cummings et al., 2010; Laissez-faire leadership, n.d.; Management by exception, n.d.; Shin & Zhou, 2003; Weberg, 2010.

Considerable research has explored the correlations between specific leadership styles and outcomes for nursing. A systematic review of the research found that transformational and relational leadership styles enhance nurse satisfaction, recruitment, and retention and foster a healthy work environment. Conversely, task-focused leadership styles correlated with lower job satisfaction, reduced effectiveness and productivity, greater emotional exhaustion, and poorer emotional health (Cummings et al., 2010). Weberg (2010) found that transformational leadership was significantly related to increased staff well-being, increased staff satisfaction, decreased burnout, and decreased overall stress in nurses. "With current nursing shortages, on the job retirement, and an uncivil mentality in health care, transformational leadership offers a tangible solution to create healthy work environments, improve staff retention and empower the bedside practitioner" (p. 257).

Transforming Your Organization

Leadership within the model of whole-person caring is transformational in nature. I use the metaphor of the diamond to demonstrate the effect that the whole-person caring model exerts on an organization. The same process that transforms each person in the organization extends to the organization's leadership culture. The process of integrating the spiritual into every aspect of our lives ultimately results in self-realization. When leadership operates from this realm, the result is an organization that is transformed and realizes its greatest potential.

The Healing Field of Management

The foundation for leadership in the WPC model is based in the spiritual or energetic realm. That means leaders intentionally access that state of consciousness and operate from that perspective. This is the same process discussed in the section about therapeutic partnering. It involves centering and getting in touch with our deepest feelings of love and caring. When we access those feelings in a centered state, we become heart centered. That doesn't mean we get all gooey and mushy. It means we are connected with the part of ourselves that is of love and compassion. We are not operating from a sense of obligation or what should be done, but we begin to ask questions such as, "What serves the greatest good in this situation?"

Managers who lead from this perspective genuinely care for and are concerned about their employees. The staff knows the manager will always be there to support them. The manager takes time to understand the staff's concerns and to really appreciate their perspective. In the model of whole-person caring, we call this the *healing field of management.* Leaders who lead with this consciousness create a work environment in which staff flourish and grow. The hospital in the case study in Chapter 4, "Integrating the Model of Whole-Person Caring," had such a manager. She exemplified what it was to be a healing presence. She was a role model and guided her staff to reach their potential. She empowered her staff to be leaders and encouraged the many patient-care and staff-care initiatives that evolved. Offering seminars, workshops, and in-services on stress management and self-care further promoted the healing environment in the hospital. The manager created the vision; through role-modeling and continually maintaining a healing field of management, the hospital culture was transformed.

Spiritual Leadership That Transforms

The metaphor of the diamond can help us understand how transformational leadership can change an organization. The metaphor gives us an image and a vision of what can evolve in our own workplace. From the perspective of the WPC model, the organization exhibits its own aspects and has its own emotional, physical, social/relational, and mental dimensions. (See Figure 9.2.)

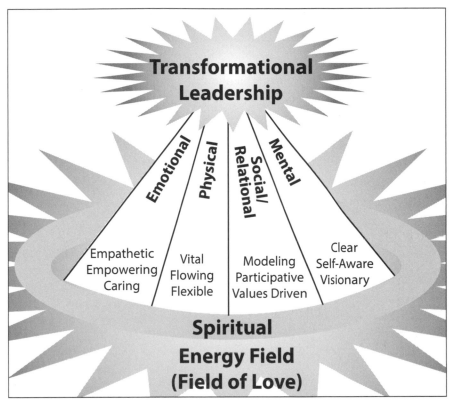

Figure 9.2   Concept of transformational leadership in the WPC model.

The spiritual or energetic realm infuses leadership with love, meaning, and respect. In the organization's emotional realm, this manifests as caring, empowering, and empathetic leadership. These are characteristics that leaders exhibit in their interactions with staff. They possess a caring and empathetic attitude, and the staff understands that the leader has their best interests at heart.

Leadership arising from spiritual values physically manifests as an organization that is flexible and flowing and that has vitality. In the WPC model, leaders are able to shift directions and change plans, and exhibit a great tendency toward innovation. Energy, ideas, and creativity flow freely at every level of the organization.

The social/relational aspect reflects a leadership style that is participatory in nature and values driven. Shared governance naturally evolves in an atmosphere in which each person is encouraged to participate in problem solving and critical thinking. Each person is empowered to take responsibility and is given the authority to make decisions related to the care they deliver. Unit problems are solved by those with the greatest expertise, and all are encouraged to participate in promoting health and healing. From the social/relational context, everyone becomes a model of leadership.

What's Love Got to Do With It?

An interesting thing happened as this model was being developed. As I was constructing the diamond figure for whole-person leadership (refer to Figure 9.2), I placed the word love in the emotional realm. After all, isn't love one of the first ways spirituality might manifest in the emotional realm of an organization? Well, as soon as I placed the word love in the emotional segment, the computer immediately kicked it out and relocated it at the foundation of the figure, just below the spiritual realm. I thought I must have mistakenly pressed the wrong key, so I tried again…and again…and again. I must have dragged the word love up into the emotional aspect at least 50 times, only to have the computer kick it down below the spiritual realm. I persisted for 2 hours, adjusting the font, increasing the size of the diamond, until I finally gave up.

In that moment of complete surrender to my computer, I realized that there was a greater message being conveyed to me. I understood that love is the basis of all that is. Love is the fundamental energy that cradles our existence. It is the glue that holds our universe together. All healing essentially comes from this field of love.

So love has everything to do with it. When we get in touch with the spiritual realm, we are infusing our lives with this infinite source of love. We are infusing our relationships, thoughts, and feelings in the greatest transformative power that exists. When we access this realm, whether it is in a leadership role or at the bedside with a patient, we are connecting with an infinite field of love that nurtures us and those around us.

Finally, from the mental perspective, transformational leadership creates a strong sense of vision and purpose with a consciousness characterized by awareness and clarity. New ways of seeing things naturally arise, and new ideas emerge from this expanded perspective. When we are anxious, our awareness narrows, and we do not see things clearly. When the heart of the organization awakens, its vision becomes clear and its mission and purpose are enlivened.

The Evolution of Leadership

Evolving toward this type of transformational leadership is an ongoing process in an organization. Leaders must learn to access their own spiritual or energetic essence to be effective. Activities that can help leaders access their spiritual nature include the following:

- Prayer
- Meditation
- Reflective and introspective practices
- Centering methods
- Journaling
- Dream work
- Learning to be fully present to life

The evolution of leadership is a process of deep inner growth, change, and development. This evolution cannot be directly communicated to others; however, it can be role-modeled, mentored, and facilitated by wise leaders. Leadership is a process of self-discovery and self-appropriated learning (Vaill, 2000).

Spirituality in leadership is a topic that has been given more attention in the last few years. Authors have identified a void—something missing in the leadership literature—and have attempted to examine how a greater sense of spirituality in the workplace might be fostered (Avolio, Walumbwa, & Weber, 2009). Some contend that spiritual leadership fosters the creation of organizational cultures characterized by altruistic love, where leaders and followers express genuine care, concern, and appreciation for both themselves and others.

> The ultimate effect of spiritual leadership is to bring together or create a sense of fusion among the four fundamental forces of human existence (body, mind, heart, and spirit) so that people are motivated for high performance, have increased organizational commitment, and personally experience joy, peace, and serenity. (Fry, 2003, p. 727)

This is precisely what the model of whole-person caring was designed to do. Spirituality is not a separate process, but it is the very foundation of our being. Our spiritual dimension is the essence of who we are. As we come closer and closer to that essence, every aspect of our lives becomes integrated and transformed. When leaders lead from this perspective, the soul of the organization emerges, and a caring and healing environment is created. Leadership development within the model of whole-person caring is a spiritual practice: transforming us, our patients, and our coworkers.

Summary

Therapeutic partnering and transformational leadership are key concepts of the model of whole-person caring. Therapeutic partnering in the WPC model is defined as a relationship between people whose common mission and purpose is to promote healing and wellness and is characterized by mutual power, respect, compassion, trust, and clear communication. There are two primary relationships involved in therapeutic partnering: the relationship between the health care provider and the patient and the relationship between health care providers.

Therapeutic partnerships promote healing and wellness. In therapeutic partnerships, the health care provider creates sacred space for the patient through the process of heart centering. This results in many positive emotional and physiological effects. In the model of whole-person caring, we call this the *field of healing*. A person who receives this type of care often experiences a deep level of caring and a feeling of being healed. The health care provider also benefits from the positive effects that are generated through the field of healing because they are an inseparable part of the energy field. This is a wonderful antidote to compassion fatigue, which is so prevalent among nurses and caregivers.

Therapeutic partnering empowers people to take control of their health. In therapeutic partnering, the patient is a partner in his or her plan of care and treatment. While the provider offers a diagnosis and options for treatment, the patient ultimately decides what he or she will do and is in control of decisions regarding his or her own health. This is paramount in reducing the incidence of chronic disease and creating a healthier society. Therapeutic partnering encourages and supports patients in developing their own practice and plans for healing and wellness.

In the workplace, therapeutic partnering fosters respect, compassion, trust, and clear communication. Every member of the team is treated equally and is crucial in providing the best possible care. Therapeutic partnering fosters a caring and healing environment in the workplace.

The concept of therapeutic partnering is particularly useful in the integrative health care setting. Integrative care involves combining conventional medicine with CAM practices. The prevailing model is based on inequitable partnerships where the medical practitioner is the gatekeeper and the CAM practitioner functions as a subordinate. The concept of therapeutic partnerships requires that care is patient focused, that collaboration takes place, and that practices will evolve based on their clinical effectiveness and without bias toward status or position.

Leadership within the model of whole-person caring is spiritually based and transformational in nature. The foundation for leadership in the WPC model is based in the spiritual or energetic realm. Leaders must learn to access their own spiritual or energetic essence to be effective. Activities that can help leaders access their spiritual nature include prayer, meditation, reflective and introspective practices, centering methods, journaling, dream work, and learning to be fully present to life. The evolution of leadership is a process of deep inner growth, change, and development. Leadership development within the model of whole-person caring is a spiritual practice, transforming us, our patients, and our coworkers.

References

Anderson, R. (2000). A case study in integrative medicine: Alternative theories and the language of biomedicine. *Journal of Alternative and Complementary Medicine, 5*(2), 165–173.

Avolio, B. J., Bass, B. M., & Jung, D. I. (1999). Re-examining the components of transformational and transactional leadership using the multifactor leadership questionnaire. *Journal of Occupational and Organizational Psychology, 72*(4), 441–462.

Avolio, B., Walumbwa, F., & Weber, T. (2009). *Leadership: Current theories, research, and future directions.* University of Nebraska-Lincoln. Management Department Faculty Publications. Paper 37. Retrieved from http://digitalcommons.unl.edu/managementfacpub/37/

Bass, B. M., & Avolio, B. J. (1994). *Improving organizational effectiveness through transformational leadership.* London, England: SAGE Publications.

Covey, S. (1992). *Principle centered leadership.* New York, NY: Fireside/Simon & Schuster.

Cummings, G., MacGregor, T., Davey, M., Lee, H., Wong, C., Lo, E.,…Stafford, E. (2010). Leadership styles and outcome patterns for the nursing workforce and work environment: A systematic review. *International Journal of Nursing Studies, 47,* 363–385.

Fry, L.W. (2003). Toward a theory of spiritual leadership. *Leadership Quarterly, 14,* 693–727.

Koloroutis, M. (2004). *Relationship-based care: A model for transforming practice.* Minneapolis, MN: Creative Healthcare Management.

Laissez-faire leadership. (n.d.) In BusinessDictionary.com. Retrieved from http://www.businessdictionary.com/definition/laissez-faire-leadership.html

Leckridge, B. (2004). The future of complementary and alternative medicine: Models of integration. *Journal of Alternative and Complementary Medicine, 10*(2), 413–416.

Management by exception. (n.d.). In BusinessDictionary.com. Retrieved from http://www.businessdictionary.com/definition/management-by-exception-MBE.html

McCraty, R., & Reese, R. (2009). *The central role of the heart in generating and sustaining positive emotions*. No. 06–022. Boulder Creek, CA: Institute of HeartMath, Publications.

Peters, D., Chaitow, L., Harris, G., & Morrison, S. (2002). *Integrating complementary therapies in primary care*. Edinburgh, Scotland: Churchill Livingstone.

Shin, S. J. & Zhou, J. (2003). Transformational leadership, conservation, and creativity: Evidence from Korea. *Academy of Management Journal, 46*(6), 703–714.

Templeman, K. & Robinson, A. (2011). Integrative medicine models in contemporary primary health care. *Complementary Therapies in Medicine, 19*(2), 84–92.

Thornton, L. (2006). *Creating a healing environment*. Fresno, CA: Self-published course manual.

Vaill, P. (2000). Reflections on time and leadership. *The Inner Edge*, December/January 1999/2000, pp. 5–6.

Weberg, D. (2010). Transformational leadership and staff retention: An evidence review with implications for healthcare systems. *Nursing Administration Quarterly, 34*(3), 246–258.

10

Caring as Sacred Practice

"The highest happiness of man…is to have
probed what is knowable and quietly to revere
what is unknowable."

–Johann Wolfgang von Goethe

In the model of whole-person caring, caring for people is considered to be sacred work. The final concept of the model, caring as sacred practice, helps evolve the attitude and approach that we bring to our work and into our lives. Transforming our workplace is first and foremost a matter of transforming ourselves. So beginning to perceive ourselves as sacred is the first step in this journey.

How do we perceive ourselves as sacred? What does it mean to do sacred work? The idea of sacred is not to be misconstrued with being religious and singing hymnals in the hallways. It is not about being sanctimonious, self-righteous, or holy (as in holier-than-thou). It does not mean that we must be somber and serious in our dealings with people or that we can't engage in activities that are fun and playful. It has nothing to do with being pompous or boring. Rather, sacred is about having a deep respect and reverence for life. It is born of an understanding that all life is precious and that all people are to be valued and treated with kindness. It comes from a deep knowingness that the purpose of our life is not simply to do our work but to do our work with great love and compassion.

Approaching our lives and work as sacred invites us to live life from our authentic self, from that place where our greatest wisdom reigns, from that place that is our divine birthright. It is about getting up in the morning and taking a moment to appreciate that we are here on Earth for another day to love, learn, and align ourselves with the creative force that expresses itself through us. It is knowing that we are here as both servants and masters—servants for the greater good and masters of our own thoughts, feelings, and emotions. Approaching our life as sacred is having a deep respect and reverence for all of life…beginning with ourselves.

Cultivating the Healer Within

Each of us has the ability to heal. It is our birthright. Some may not choose to connect with that potential, but for all of us, it is there. Healing happens when we access the ground of our being, the essence of our self, and allow our consciousness to rest in that infinite space. Sound easy? It really isn't difficult. It isn't magical, and it isn't mysterious. It just involves getting in touch with who we are!

Anyone who has been in a relationship with another knows that this process doesn't happen in one night over dinner and a bottle of wine. It may take a lifetime to get to know and to accept another. The paradox is that we must know ourselves before we can be in a healthy relationship with anyone else. We must learn to accept and love who we are before we can accept and love another.

Getting to know ourselves is a gradual process of uncovering the many layers that have shrouded us from our true self. It is a process much like peeling an onion. With each layer, we come closer and closer to the center—and like peeling an onion, the process can bring us to tears. There are many different practices that we can use to develop a closer relationship with ourselves—many paths to our true self.

Meditation

Meditation is perhaps the single most useful reflective practice to help gain self-awareness and self-knowledge, increase intuition, and enhance one's spiritual development. Because self-awareness, self-knowledge, and intuition are foundational to creating a caring-healing presence, meditating regularly is an important practice (Thornton & Mariano, 2013).

Meditation has been used for centuries to increase calmness and physical relaxation, improve psychological balance, cope with illness, and enhance overall health and well-being. The literature on meditation suggests that it is a very powerful tool for learning to control our attention, regulate our emotions, and increase our self-awareness (Briggs, 2010). Recent studies suggest that meditation activates various parts in the brain, particularly the amygdala, a region associated with processing emotion (Briggs, 2012).

Meditation is practiced in many ways and forms: mantra meditation, breathing meditation, chakra meditation, mindfulness meditation, walking meditation, kundalini meditation, kriya yoga meditation, and Christian meditation, to name a few. Some of the more popular forms of meditation are mindfulness meditation, sitting meditation, qigong, and heart meditation. Meditation practices are often rooted in spiritual practices, but many people practice meditation outside of a religious context. As cited in Briggs, the 2007 National Health Interview Survey revealed that some 20 million U.S. adults use meditation for health purposes (2010).

Common Forms of Meditation

- Mindfulness, also called *vipassana,* comes from the Buddhist tradition. Mindfulness is likely the most popular form of meditation in the Western world. It's all about "being present," letting your mind run, and accepting whatever thoughts come up while practicing detachment from each thought. Mindfulness is taught along with awareness of the breath, though the breathing is often considered to be just one sensation among many others, not a particular focus.

- Zazen is the generic term for seated meditation in the Buddhist tradition, but in the modern Zen tradition, it is often referred to as "just sitting." It is a minimal kind of meditation, done for long periods of time, with little instruction beyond the basics of posture (sit with your back straight). There is no particular attention to the breath or an attempt to change the breath. Zazen is the "anti-method" approach to meditation, but it is often done in conjunction with a concentration on a certain aspect of Buddhist scripture or a paradoxical sentence, story, or question, called a *koan.*

- Transcendental meditation (TM) is a simplified practice that emerges from Vedanta, the meditative tradition within Hinduism. In TM, you sit with your back straight (ideally in the lotus or half-lotus posture) and use a mantra, a sacred word that is repeated. Your focus is on rising above all that is impermanent.

- Qigong is a form of Taoist meditation that uses the breath to circulate energy through the organs and energy centers of the body in an oval pattern called the *microcosmic orbit.* Attention is focused on the breath and the circulation of energy (called *qi* or *chi*). Attention is also focused on the three major centers used in Taoist meditation: a point about two inches below the navel, the center of the chest, and the center of the forehead. Qigong uses the breath to direct energy and to circulate energy in the body and spirit.

- Heart rhythm meditation (HRM) focuses on the breath and heartbeat, making the breath full, deep, rich, rhythmic, and balanced. Attention is focused on the heart as the center of the energetic system. In HRM, the person identifies with the heart. Focusing on the breath, the field emanating from the heart is sent to different parts of the body and then out into the subtle energy field. This is a practice that energizes the body and moves the consciousness toward self-awareness and self-compassion. (See Appendix C, "Meditation on the Heart.")

Excerpted and revised with permission from Bair, 2010.

Meditation is a quiet turning inward. It is the practice of focusing one's attention internally to achieve clearer consciousness and inner stillness. Meditation allows a better understanding of the self and increased receptivity to insights arising from one's deeper being. Dan Benor, MD, says the following about meditation (personal communication, May 17, 2011):

> Meditation is healing in and of itself. Meditation is a gateway into spiritual awareness and healing. By quieting our mind, we can access dimensions in which spiritual healing can occur. Meditation allows us to quiet the mind from its chatter and its focus on everyday, outer-world matters. It helps us open into transcendent awareness.

John Kabat-Zinn (1994), a teacher of mindfulness meditation, describes his practice in the following way:

> It has everything to do with waking up and living in harmony with oneself and with the world. It has to do with examining who we are, with questioning our view of the world and our place in it, and with cultivating some appreciation for the fullness of each moment we are alive. Most of all, it has to do with being in touch. (p. 3)

There are a variety of approaches in meditation. Hopefully, there is one that will resonate with you. The basic steps of meditation are laid out in the upcoming sidebar. This can be a starting point, although after 30-some years of meditating, I still gravitate toward this basic approach.

Basic Steps of Meditation

1. Pick a focus word or phrase or prayer.

2. Sit quietly in a meditative position.

   - Sit up so your spine is erect. Use a straight-backed chair or sit on the floor or a sofa with pillows to support your back.

   - Find a place to meditate where you will not be interrupted. Designate a special spot in your home or work area to create a space where you can more easily become relaxed.

3. Close your eyes.

4. Focus your attention and internal gaze at the point between your eyebrows, sometimes referred to as the "third eye."

5. Relax your body.

   - Mentally scan your body for areas of tension. Breathe into those areas to release the tension.

   - It is a good idea to do stretching exercises, yoga, or a progressive muscle relaxation before sitting down to meditate. Focus on stretching the back and neck muscles so that your body is free from any tension, which will be distracting.

6. Breathe slowly and naturally and, as you do, repeat your focus word as you exhale.

   - Sometimes repeating a word on inhalation and then a word on exhalation creates a very relaxing state. For instance, the Sanskrit words *So hum* ("I am that") are a common phrase in meditation. On the inhalation, silently repeat "So," and on the exhalation silently repeat, "Hum."

7. When any thoughts come to mind, gently refocus your attention to the point between your eyebrows and repeat the phrase with the natural rhythm of your breathing.

8. Practice the technique for 10 to 20 minutes once or twice daily.

9. Be patient and don't judge.

   - When you first begin to meditate, start with 5-minute sessions and then increase to 10 minutes over a couple of weeks.

   - Don't judge your meditation as good or bad. Don't become discouraged if your mind continues to wander. Gently refocus your attention on your phrase and breathing.

10. Set your intention for the day.
  ✒ After you have finished meditating, set an intention for the day that will help guide your thoughts, feelings, and actions, such as "I will move through the day with grace and ease. I meet all challenges with confidence, compassion, wisdom, and clarity."

Source: Thornton & Gold, 2000.

You can also practice the loving-kindness meditation discussed in Chapter 6, "Self-Compassion, Self-Care, and Self-Healing." Yet another lovely meditation is the meditation on the heart in Appendix C. There are hundreds of different meditations and meditation techniques that can help you to relax and gain access to your infinite self. Exploring different types of meditation practices will help you find one that resonates with you. Some people have a very difficult time sitting still and prefer to do a walking meditation. There are abundant resources on the Internet for you to access as well as some resource sites recommended in Appendix D, "Resources," under "Meditation Resources."

It is most important that you engage in some type of practice that enables you to quiet your mind and listen to your innermost self. When I first began meditating, I had a horrible time sitting still. My mind would incessantly wander, skipping from one idea to the next. A meditation teacher once said that the mind is like a drunken monkey; in the beginning, that is exactly what it felt like. I remember asking a meditation teacher what the difference was between prayer and meditation. The reply was simple: "When you pray, you are talking to God, and when you meditate, God is talking to you." Meditation has been a wonderful practice to gain deeper insight into who I am and to connect with that place of knowingness, love, and compassion. It is not easy at first. Be persistent, make a commitment to practice, and it will become a significant part of your life.

Reflective and Introspective Practice and Approaches

Socrates said, "The unexamined life is not worth living" (Plato, n.d.). Setting aside time each day to reflect on the activities and interactions of our day is an important practice. This is the process that allows us to learn about ourselves, our patterns, and how our behaviors affect others. It helps us live more consciously, with a greater appreciation and understanding of how our behaviors affect others and how we are affected by those around us.

Meditation is a reflective process that provides us with important insights related to deeply embedded patterns that exist in our life. An effective way of reflecting on a situation is to bring to mind the situation during your meditation. Simply ask your higher self, "What is it that I need to learn or know from this situation/interaction/problem?" Then just be aware of what comes to mind and listen with your whole being. You will be surprised at some of the profound insights that will arise in this process.

Journaling is another reflective process that we can use to give ourselves insight and provide perspective. Through journaling, self-awareness and self-understanding are enhanced and become a means of caring for oneself, as well as creating a heightened sense of responsibility in caring for others (Charles, 2010). Journaling can give us insights into the patterns of our lives and enable us to see what situations and people in our lives create positive and negative responses. Our patterns of behavior become apparent in a written record. When people journal to get in touch with their deepest thoughts and feelings, it can measurably improve physical and mental health (Pennebaker, 1990).

Reflective practices are not only techniques and methods that we use in moments of solitude; ideally, these practices become a process that occurs during our interactions. The more we learn to engage our spiritual, transcendent essence in our interactions, the more we simultaneously engage in reflection. The processes of centering, being fully present, and creating a field of healing generate a transcendent awareness that is reflective in nature. Likewise, the process of engaging our observer, discussed in Chapter 6, allows us to reflect on situations as they happen and to respond from a place of clarity without reflexively engaging in past patterns.

There are a variety of reflective approaches and practices that we can bring into our lives and work that can help us live more consciously. Incorporating reflective practices can be very challenging, however—especially in the stressful conditions inherent in health care settings and life in general. Sometimes it is useful and necessary to retreat for a weekend to rest and reflect. Incorporating an annual weekend for reflection, rest, and meditation is a wonderful way to restore and revitalize our spirit. Creating more time for reflection often gives rise to insights and understanding that we cannot achieve while immersed in our daily routines.

Dream Work

Dreams have been explored since ancient times for prophecy and divination. The ancient Egyptians believed that dreams were messages from the gods. The Greeks had sacred places for dream incubation and would induce sleep through herbal concoctions to elicit dreams that would help them to treat various diseases and afflictions. The Zulu people of South Africa regard dreams as messages from their ancestors (Dream Interpretation Dictionary, 2011). Many people believe that we can access other dimensions in our sleep and gain valuable insights through these interdimensional connections.

The work of Jung has helped us grasp the powerful role dreams can play in understanding ourselves. The symbols, premonitions, and metaphors that we receive from the subconscious mind can give us powerful insights about our lives. "The dream shows the inner truth and reality of the patient as it really is: not as I conjecture it to be, and not as he would like it to be, but as it is" (Jung, 1985, p. 304).

Dreams are often cryptic and may represent parts of ourselves that we have repressed and are not conscious of. Over time, and with the practice of writing and reflecting on dreams, we can develop skill in interpreting the symbols and metaphors that arise (Levin & Reich, 2013).

Tip

If you do not have many dreams and would like to increase the frequency of your dreaming, taking some vitamin B6 may help, as advised by Dr. Evarts Loomis, MD, one of the founders of the American Holistic Medical Association (personal communication, July 2002).

Keeping a dream journal is one of the best ways to become proficient in interpreting your dreams. Here are some basic guidelines:

- Keep the journal next to your bed so you can record your dream upon awakening.

- When you awaken, remain in the same position to remember your dream. This engages your body memory (Levin & Reich, 2013).

- Write down any information that might help you understand your dream. Include such things as what time you went to bed, whether you took any medication, what TV program you were watching or what you were reading or doing before you went to bed, and any significant events that occurred during the previous day.

- Include any strong feelings that you associate with the symbols in your dream.

- ◂ Write your dreams in the present tense as if you're still dreaming. This helps you remember your dreams more vividly.

- ◂ Review your journal periodically to see what themes have been unfolding.

Sometimes telling our dream to someone gives us insight. When we give voice to the dream and actually hear it, we often gain insights that we hadn't obtained by writing or just thinking about the dream.

Cultivating the healer within is a process of increasing our self-knowledge and self-awareness. This is a process that must be accompanied with great patience, kindness, love, and compassion. It is not about doing anything, but simply about resting in the essence of who we are. All the practices described are merely tools to help our busy minds let go of all the silly little thoughts that keep us from seeing our true nature. We all get glimpses of that magnificent nature in our lives. It may be through meditation, deep prayer, dreams, or a walk in the park. When we fully open our hearts to ourselves, we understand that love is the essence of who we are. It is this love that heals; it is this love that makes us whole.

Being a Healing Presence: Creating a Field of Healing

Our presence is one of the most powerful tools for healing. Realizing that we are fields of energy that are infinite and open has many implications for our practice. When we understand that there is no separation between who we are and our environment, we begin to understand the effects that our state of being can have on another. The degree to which we can be a healing presence is determined by our self-knowledge and the health and wholeness that we embrace in our own lives.

Practices such as meditation, prayer, and reflection help us access our spiritual essence and come to a greater awareness of who we are. The use of practices such as guided imagery, affirmations, and breathing techniques, to name a few, can help us create healthier ways of responding to stressful situations and bring peace and equanimity into our lives. Bringing healing practices such as massage, reflexology, acupressure, and subtle energy healing (therapeutic touch, healing touch, Reiki) into our lives helps balance and revitalize our subtle energy bodies and physical bodies. Developing healthy habits in the way we eat, sleep, breathe, and move is important to nurture our physical selves. We can nurture our hearts by bringing healthy relationships into our lives, learning to love ourselves and others, and creating therapeutic partnerships with our coworkers and patients. Expressing our creativity, believing in ourselves, and having a positive attitude and problem-solving orientation to life—these are all things that nurture our mind. There are a variety of approaches and tools that we can use to help us realize our wholeness and heal ourselves. If we want to be a healing presence in this world, we must care for and nurture all the aspects of our being. There are several practices that we can integrate into our daily work routines that can help us be a healing presence. These practices are used by healers and are also a part of the holistic nursing process.

Creating Intention

Creating an intention is a process that sets into motion what we want to manifest. McKivergen (2009) defines intent as "the conscious alignment with creative essence and divine purpose that allows the highest good to flow through a healing intervention or through life itself" (p. 722). When we align our thoughts with our creative essence, our spiritual self, then we have aligned ourselves with an infinite source of energy. While creating an intention may seem innocuous, the power of this process is enormous.

Recent research helps shed light on why this process is so dynamic. Research in the field of psychoneuroimmunology has demonstrated the effects that thoughts have on our physiology (see Chapter 7, "Self-Care and Self-Healing Practices," in the section "The Power of Thoughts and Emotions"). Creating an intentional thought not only affects our physiology, but it also affects the physical world. Tiller (2009) demonstrated that conscious intent can be imprinted in materials that can be shipped to a distant laboratory, and the intentional effect that is imprinted on them can be brought out. Recent advances in theoretical physics suggest that the space between atoms and molecules is not inert. Tiller and Dibble (2009) speculate that this vacuum may be where the intent is imprinted. Our thoughts actually carry energy that affects us physiologically and also affects our physical world. As Ralph Waldo Emerson (1867) once said, "Great men are they who see that spiritual thought is stronger than any material force, that thoughts rule the world."

Creating intentions throughout the day can help us consciously create a healing environment. For example:

- Before you get out of bed, you can create the intention, "I will have a productive day at work and have ample energy and vitality throughout the day."

- Before going into a meeting, you can create the intention, "I will communicate my thoughts with clarity, and my recommendations will be graciously received."

- Before entering a patient's room, you can create the intention, "I will be fully present for this patient and create a space where healing occurs."

Creating an intention is a powerful way for the health care provider to create a healing environment. It is a positive affirmation that aligns us with our creative force and sets into motion the caring-healing process.

Simple Centering

Centering is a process that affects our psychological, emotional, mental, and physiological being. It is a process that creates a caring-healing environment by helping us set aside our concerns and focus on the person to whom we are relating or for whom we are caring. Centering has been defined as "a calm and focused sense of self-relatedness that can be thought of as a place of inner being, a place of quietude within oneself where one feels integrated and focused" (Jackson & Latini, 2013, p.417). Slater (2013) describes a physiological effect of centering: "Centering is an altered state of consciousness that results in the centered person's hands emitting measurable extra-low frequency magnetic pulses of 0.3–3.0 hertz (Hz) that is, cycles per second" (p. 751).

There are various techniques that can be used to help a person become centered. All of the techniques involve a person's conscious intent to quiet the mind and to become focused on the here and now. Focusing on the breath is a mechanism that allows the person to set aside his or her own thoughts and feelings and become present to the moment. Using an affirmation such as, "I am here for the greater good; I give my full attention to the here and now," is also useful in the centering process. Using environmental cues to help us remember to center is also useful. Stepping through the doorway of a patient's room or using the ring of a phone as as a signal to center are some cues that can remind us to become centered before engaging in an interaction or conversation.

As cited in Macrae, Dora Kunz recommended that nurses take a moment to center themselves before any patient contact. (Dora Kunz and Delores Krieger developed therapeutic touch [TT] and introduced TT into nursing.) Kunz recommended further that in the half minute that you take to wash your hands between patients, you do the following (Macrae, 2001):

1. Take a deep breath.

2. Quiet your mind using mental focus.

3. Think of the tension flowing out of you and going down the drain.

Heart Centering

Heart centering involves the process of simple centering along with consciously connecting to feelings of love and compassion. Heart centering and intention setting are two practices in which the holistic nurse engages prior to patient interaction. In this process, the health care provider sets asides concerns and thoughts, focuses his or her attention on the heart, and connects with feelings of love and compassion. The technique is as follows:

1. Pause for a moment before entering the patient's room.

2. Set aside any concerns regarding the past or the future. These can be picked up when leaving the room.

3. Gently close your eyes.

4. Breathe deeply and slowly.

5. Repeat to yourself, "I am here for the greater good of this patient. I give my full attention to the here and now."

6. Direct awareness to the area around your heart, bringing to mind something or someone that evokes your love and compassion.

7. When connected with that feeling of love and compassion, repeat, "I am present to the moment."

This entire process should take only between 10 to 20 seconds. You have now created a field of healing.

Imagine how it would feel if everyone in our work environment communicated from a place of love and compassion. How would that be different from what we presently experience? It doesn't take more time, and it doesn't require more money. It is the simple act of quieting our minds by setting aside our concerns and mental chatter and allowing our consciousness to rest in the ground of our being—that place of knowingness, love, and compassion. It doesn't require us to do anything. It simply requires that we connect with who we really are.

Being heart centered results in a physiological state called *heart coherence.* Heart coherence—also referred to as physiologic coherence, cardiac coherence, or resonance—is a functional mode measured by heart rate variability (HRV) analysis, wherein a person's heart rhythm pattern becomes ordered. Research has demonstrated that heart centering and its resultant heart coherence creates many positive physiological and psychological effects, as presented in the upcoming sidebar.

Heart coherence may help to connect people with their intuitive inner guidance. Research suggests that the heart's energy field (energetic heart) is coupled with a field of information that is not bound by the classic limits of time and space. This evidence comes from a rigorous experimental study that investigated the proposition that the body receives and processes information about a future event before the event actually happens (McCraty, Atkinson, & Bradley, 2004). McCraty and Childre explain that the intuitive heart, or heart intelligence, is coupled with a deeper part of oneself—what some may call their higher power or their higher capacities. When we are heart centered and coherent, we have a tighter coupling and closer alignment with our deeper source of intuitive intelligence (McCraty & Childre, 2010).

Effects of Heart Coherence

Some effects of heart coherence include the following:

- It balances heart rhythms.
- It increases IgA (immunoglobulin A) levels and natural killer cell levels.
- It increases mental clarity and problem solving.
- It reduces sleeplessness, body aches, and fatigue.
- It reduces anger, sadness, hypertension, and other chronic problems.
- It may help people connect with inner intuitive guidance.

Sources: McCraty, Atkinson, & Bradley, 2004; McCraty & Reese, 2009; McCraty & Childre, 2010.

Research also shows that the positive mental and physiologic effects experienced by the health care provider can be transmitted to the patient. When a person maintains a coherent electromagnetic field through the process of centering, that person's energy field positively affects those in the surrounding environment. Morris (2010) reports that a coherent energy field can be generated and/or enhanced by the intention of small groups of participants trained to send coherence-facilitating intentions to a target receiver.

It is also believed that information about a person's emotional state is encoded in the heart's electromagnetic field and is communicated into the external environment (McCraty & Childre, 2010). When the health care provider becomes heart centered, a healing environment is created in which the person feels safe, nurtured, and loved and is in an optimal state for healing to occur.

Transcendent/Transpersonal Presence

Presence has been defined as a way of being, relating, being with, and being there. These perspectives each speak to different facets of the quality and characteristics of the attention that one person gives to another in a relationship (Thornton & Mariano, 2013).

Osterman and Schwartz-Barcott (1996) describe four types of presence. This categorization is a good teaching tool to help us identify at what level we are relating to people. Most likely, we move through each level throughout the day. The four types of presence are as follows:

- **Presence:** In this type of presence, one is physically present but self-absorbed. There is no interaction. This reduces stress in that there is reassurance that someone is there. It may be quieting and restorative. However, there is no personal engagement, and there is often missed communication.

- **Partial presence:** In this type of presence, one is physically present but is focused on mechanical or technical issues rather than on others. This reduces stress and may solve a mechanical problem, but there is no interpersonal connectedness.

- **Full presence:** With this type of presence, one is physically present and attentive, making eye contact, leaning in. The person is psychologically present, displaying attentive listening behavior, focused on another, interactive. Essential communication is occurring, along with the solving of a human problem and/or relief of here-and-now distress. While much of this is positive, this may be too much energy for the recipient or may feel negative to a recipient.

- **Transcendent presence:** With this type of presence, one is physically and psychologically present, even holistic. The focus of energy is centered. The person is transcending, oriented beyond here and now, sustaining while at the same time transforming reality. This state of being involves a high degree of skilled communication, love, and human caring. It decreases loneliness. There is an expansion of consciousness, spiritual peace, hope, and meaning. A nice feeling is generated in the environment. This may result in a fusion and possible loss of objective reality and the danger of taking on the recipient's problems.

It is at the transcendent level of presence that the potential for the deepest healing occurs. Transcendent presence is transforming and more spiritual in quality, moving beyond the interactional to the transpersonal. According to Osterman and Schwartz-Barcott (1996):

> The energy in this way of presence comes from a spiritual source initiated by centering. The energy goes beyond the two people interacting and is dissipated into the environment and felt by others. Transcendent presence is felt as peaceful, comforting, and harmonious…While full presence is reality anchoring, transcendent presence sustains a person experiencing a painful reality. It is more than the use of self, although the self is important. There are no boundaries, and as such there are no limitations imposed by role. In this light, transcendent presence is more than the therapeutic use of self. The nurse recognizes the transcendent presence when a oneness is felt with the patient. (p. 28)

Watson helps us understand the sacred nature of caring in her articulation of the transpersonal caring relationship. Engaging with another at the transpersonal level involves the ability to access one's higher self and move from that place of higher consciousness in interaction with another. This process calls forth the full use of self (Watson, 1999, p. 69):

> The nurse is able to form a union with the other person on a level that transcends the physical, and that preserves the subjectivity and physicality of persons without reducing them to the moral of objects.…The union of feelings can potentiate self-healing and discovery in his or her own existence. That is the great attractive force of the art of transpersonal caring in nursing. (Watson, 1999, p. 68)

The descriptions of transcendent presence and the transpersonal caring relationship help us understand what caring as sacred practice means. Our ability to embody transcendent/transpersonal presence is the result of experience and engaging in processes of deep reflection and inquiry. The practices of creating intention and becoming heart centered are useful tools to help us create a field of healing. When we are able to connect with our own heart and soul, we can establish that connection with others.

Honoring the Wholeness of Life

In honoring a person's wholeness, our efforts are geared toward promoting healing, unity, and harmony. The wholeness of life is woven into a sacred tapestry—and in this light, all life is sacred. To be in the right relationship with life requires that we acknowledge *all* of life.

Embracing the wholeness and sacredness of life involves being present to all of life. This means being present to that which we may perceive to be good and that which we may perceive to be bad. It is staying present to those situations that bring us happiness and those that bring us sorrow. It involves being present to those relationships that bring us peace of mind and those that create inner turmoil.

Being present to all of life may not be pleasant and may not feel healing. At times, being fully present to life may feel uncomfortable, deeply disturbing, and even painful. However, staying present and connecting with someone center to center, whether bearing witness to their joy, their suffering, their grief, their torment, or their confusion, creates a healing environment and honors the wholeness of their life.

In the model of whole-person caring, caring for people is sacred work. As health care providers, how we choose to relate and interact matters greatly. Health care workers have a responsibility to create and hold a loving, sacred space for patients. The model of whole-person caring reminds us that caring for people is an honor and a privilege.

Summary

The final concept of the model of whole-person caring, caring as sacred practice, helps evolve the attitude and approach that we bring to our work and into our lives. Approaching our life as sacred means having a deep respect and reverence for all of life…beginning with ourselves.

Each of us has the ability to heal. Healing is a process involving self-knowledge and self-awareness. Reflective practices facilitate the process of self-knowledge and self-awareness and therefore help to cultivate our inner healer. Meditation is perhaps the single most useful reflective practice to help gain self-awareness and self-knowledge, increase intuition, and enhance one's spiritual development. Journaling is another reflective process that enhances self-understanding. Dream work can provide insights on those dimensions of ourselves that we have repressed or shut down.

Being reflective while we are interacting with others is achieved through centering, transpersonal/transcendent communication, and other practices such as engaging our observer. These practices allow us to reflect on situations as they happen and to respond from a place of clarity, without reflexively engaging past patterns.

Our presence is one of the most powerful tools for healing. Realizing that we are open fields of energy that are in continual process with everything else helps us understand the effects that our state of being can have on another. All that we are—our thoughts, behaviors, emotions, that which is conscious, and that which is unconscious—interacts and affects everything and everyone in our environment. The degree to which we can be a healing presence is in large part determined by our self-knowledge and the health and wholeness that we embrace in our own lives.

Creating a field of healing is facilitated through intention, heart centering, and transcendent/transpersonal presence. Creating an intention is a powerful way for the health care provider to create a healing environment. It is a positive affirmation that aligns us with our creative force and sets into motion the caring-healing process.

Heart centering is a process in which the health care provider sets asides concerns and thoughts, focuses his or her attention on the heart, and connects with feelings of love and compassion. This creates a condition in the heart called *heart coherence* that results in many physiological changes, such as increased IgA levels, balanced heart rhythms, and increased mental clarity. In addition, heart coherence reduces sleeplessness, body aches, and fatigue, and reduces anger, sadness, hypertension, and other chronic problems. When the health care provider becomes heart centered, a healing environment is created in which the patient feels safe, nurtured, and loved, and is in an optimal state for healing to occur.

Presence is defined as a way of being, a way of relating, a way of being with, and a way of being there. Research has identified four ways of being: presence, partial presence, full presence, and transcendent presence. It is at the transcendent level of presence that the potential for the deepest healing occurs. The transpersonal caring relationship is similar to transcendent presence. Transcendent presence is felt as peaceful, comforting, and harmonious. When we are able to connect with our own heart and soul, we can establish that connection with others.

Embracing the wholeness and sacredness of life involves being present to all of life. Staying present and connecting with someone center to center, whether bearing witness to their joy, their suffering, their grief, their torment, or their confusion, is a type of presence that creates a healing environment and honors the wholeness of that person's life.

References

Bair, A. (2010). 8 basic kinds of meditation (and why you should meditate on your heart). *Institute for Applied Meditation*. Retrieved from http://www.iam-u.org/index.php/8-basic-kinds-of-meditation-and-why-you-should-meditate-on-your-heart

Briggs, J. (2010). *Exploring the power of meditation*. National Center for Complementary and Alternative Medicine (NCCAM). Retrieved from http://nccam.nih.gov/about/offices/od/2010-06.htm

Briggs, J. (2012). *New research on meditation—It's all about the brain*. National Center for Complementary and Alternative Medicine (NCCAM). Retrieved from https://nccam.nih.gov/research/blog/portfolio

Charles, J. (2010). Journaling: Creating space for "I". *Creative Nursing, 16*(4), 180–184.

Dream Interpretation Dictionary. (2011). *History of dream interpretation*. Retrieved from http://www.dreaminterpretation-dictionary.com

Emerson, R.W. (1867). *Progress of culture*. Address read before the Phi Beta Kappa Society at Cambridge on July 18, 1867. Retrieved from: http://www.rwe.org/complete-works/viii---letters-and-social-aims/progress-of-culture.html

Jackson, C., & Latini, C. (2013). Touch and hand-mediated therapies. In B. Dossey and L. Keegan (Eds.). *Holistic nursing: A hand-book for practice* (6th ed.) (pp. 417–437). Burlington, MA: Jones and Bartlett Learning.

Jung, C. (1985). *The practice of psychotherapy: Essays on the psychology of the transference and other subjects* (2nd ed.). Princeton, NJ: Princeton University Press.

Kabat-Zinn, J. (1994). *Wherever you go there you are*. New York, NY: Hyperion.

Levin, J. D., & Reich, J. L. (2013). Self-reflection. In B. Dossey & L. Keegan (Eds.). *Holistic nursing: A hand-book for practice* (6th ed.) (pp. 247–260). Burlington, MA: Jones & Bartlett Learning.

Macrae, J. (2001). *Nursing as a spiritual practice: A contemporary application of Florence Nightingale's views*. New York, NY: Springer Publishing Company.

McCraty, R., & Reese, R. (2009). *The central role of the heart in generating and sustaining positive emotions*. Institute of HeartMath, Publication No. 06-022. Boulder Creek, CA: HeartMath Research Center.

McCraty, R., & Childre, D. (2010). Coherence: Bridging personal, social, and global health. *Alternative Therapies, 16*(4), 10–24.

McCraty, R., Atkinson, M., & Bradley, R.T. (2004). Electrophysiological evidence of intuition: Part 1. The surprising role of the heart. *Journal of Alternative and Complementary Medicine, 10*(1), 133–143.

McKivergin, M. (2009). The nurse as an instrument of healing. In B. Dossey and L. Keegan (Eds.). *Holistic nursing: A hand-book for practice* (5th ed.) (pp. 721–737). Sudbury, MA: Jones and Bartlett.

Morris, S. (2010). Achieving collective coherence: Group effects on heart rate variability coherence and heart rhythm synchronization. *Alternative Therapies, 16*(4), 62–72.

Osterman, P., & Schwartz-Barcott, D. (1996). Presence: Four ways of being there. *Nursing Forum, 31*(2), 23–30. Retrieved from DOI:10.1111/j.1744-6198.1996.tb00490.x

Pennebaker, J. (1990). *Opening up: The healing power of confiding in others.* New York, NY: William Morrow.

Plato. (n.d.). *Apology.* Translated by Benjamin Jowett. *Project Gutenberg.* Retrieved from http://www.gutenberg.org/files/1656/1656-h/1656-h.htm

Slater, V. (2013). Energy healing. In B. Dossey and L. Keegan (Eds.). *Holistic nursing: A hand-book for practice* (6th ed.) (pp. 751–774). Burlington, MA: Jones and Bartlett Learning.

Thornton, L. & Gold, J. (2000). *Creating a healing culture: Course I—Whole-person caring.* Roseland, NJ: Self-published workbook.

Thornton, L., & Mariano, C. (2013). Evolving from therapeutic to holistic communication. In B. Dossey & L. Keegan (Eds.), *Holistic nursing: A hand-book for practice* (6th ed.) (pp. 619–632). Burlington, MA: Jones & Bartlett Learning.

Tiller, W., & Dibble, W. (2009). A brief introduction to intention-host device research. White paper. William A. Tiller Foundation. Retrieved from http://www.tiller.org

Watson, J. (1999). *Nursing: Human science and human care, a theory of nursing.* Sudbury, MA: NLN Press/Jones and Bartlett.

A

Integration of Organizational Values

Research at Hospital in Case Study

The nursing management of the hospital discussed in the case study in Chapter 4, "Integrating the Model of Whole-Person Caring," wanted to determine whether the incorporation of the model of whole-person caring would have any measurable effects on employees' integration of organizational values. An educational program was designed to help participants understand and integrate the concepts of whole-person caring into their lives and work. The educational program, the transformational health care leadership course, consisted of an initial 2-day seminar followed by a 6-month course of study, culminating with a 2-day seminar.

A research study was designed and conducted to determine the effects that the transformational health care leadership course had on participants' integration of organizational values. Participants were tested prior to taking the course, immediately after completing the course, and 6 months following the completion of the course. Data supported that the transformational health care leadership course positively affected the integration of organizational values. The research was prepared and conducted by Dr. Debra Topham.

Data Collection and Instrumentation

Prior to participation in the transformational leadership course, course participants completed a demographic form and the self-report inventory (SRI), which measured the extent to which the respondents had integrated organizational values into their practice.

Nurse managers at the hospital constructed the self-reporting inventory, establishing content validity. Input was obtained from facilitators of the transformational leadership course and the data analysis person. Instrument reliability was established via internal consistency. The SRI was found to have an alpha coefficient of .86, an acceptable level of reliability.

A total of 20 participants and 20 control-group members submitted the SRI pre-test, mid-test, and post-test. Data was analyzed using an analysis of variance (ANOVA) to test differences between participant and control-group mean scores. There were no significant differences between the participant-group and control-group mean scores on any of the pre-tests, mid-tests, or post-tests. Therefore, the data for both groups was combined to analyze differences between pre-test, mid-test, and post-test scores.

This is consistent with the theoretical framework for the project. According to Martha Rogers, the human energy field is integral with the environmental energy field, and, as such, they are in constant mutual process. Therefore, what affects the human energy field will also affect its environment, including other human energy fields. Based on Rogers's theory, it could be anticipated that as participants of the transformational leadership course integrate organizational values, they would also influence the values of others in the work environment.

Data Analysis of Organizational Values

Data was analyzed for the 40 respondents completing all components of the SRI surveys. Organizational values were reflected in scores on the SRI. A composite score was computed for values representing excellence, respect, service, and teamwork. A total composite value score was also calculated, and data were analyzed for the composite value score. With the exception of teamwork, all values scores, including the overall values score, raised consistently and significantly from the pre-test to post-test, including from pre-test to mid-test. Scores rose slightly for all values, except teamwork, from the mid-test to post-test. (See Table A.1.)

Table A.1   Group Means for Test Scores

	Excellence	Honesty	Respect	Service	Teamwork	Overall Values
Pre-test mean	3.8	4.31	4.18	3.85	4.07	4.07
Mid-test mean	3.94	4.56	4.26	4.27	4.57	4.3
Post-test mean	4.05	4.63	4.45	4.29	4.24	4.36

As stated, the change in scores from pre-test to post-test was statistically significant, except for the value of teamwork. Paired t-tests were run to compare pre-test and post-test scores, pre-test and mid-test scores, and mid-test and post-test scores. The overall values score, excellence value, honesty value, respect value, and service value showed a statistically significant increase from pre-test to post-test scores. Further analysis revealed that the increase between pre-test and mid-test scores was most statistically significant. (See Table A.2.)

Table A.2 T-Test Scores for Pre-Test, Mid-Test, and Post-Test Means

	Pre-Test/Post-Test	Pre-Test/Mid-Test	Mid-Test/Post-Test
Overall values	t = 3.89, p = .001*	t = 4.34, p = .000*	t = 0.68, p = .053
Excellence	t = 2.65, p = .014*	t = 3.86, p = .001*	t = 0.69, p = .496
Honesty	t = 2.77, p = .011*	t = 2.35, p = .026**	t = 0.37, p = .715
Respect	t = 3.14, p = .005*	t = 1.47, p = .153	t = 1.91, p = .070
Service	t = 3.52, p = .002*	t = 2.59, p = .015**	t = 1.10, p = .285
Teamwork	t = 1.02, p = .316	t = 2.07, p = .047**	t = −1.13, p = .269

*= significant at the .01 level, ** = significant at the .05 level*

Results

Data supports that the transformational leadership course positively influenced the integration of organizational values in persons responding on the SRI. This influence was most significant between the pre-test and mid-test scores. The mid-test point coincided with completion of the transformational leadership course. A continuing shift in the integration of organizational values, as measured by post-test scores, speaks to the ongoing benefits of the transformational leadership course 6 months after its completion.

The lack of significant change in the teamwork scores and the mid-test to post-test drop in teamwork scores can be attributed to many factors. In this organization, the time after the mid-test data collection point was when two different hospital campuses were merged into one campus. It takes time for workers to re-establish work teams and develop trust with coworkers. It is anticipated that these scores will go up.

B

Loving-Kindness Meditation for Beginners

Set aside 20 to 40 minutes for the purpose of bringing warmth and goodwill into your life. To begin, sit in a comfortable position, reasonably upright and relaxed. Close your eyes fully or partially. Take a few deep breaths to settle into your body and into the present moment. Then do the following:

1. Put your hands over your heart to remind yourself that you are bringing not only attention, but also loving attention, to your experience. Feel the warmth of your hands, the gentle pressure of your hands, and feel how your chest rises and falls beneath your hands with every breath.

2. Bring to mind a person or other living being who naturally makes you smile. This could be a child, your grandmother, your cat or dog—whoever naturally brings happiness to your heart. Perhaps it's a bird outside your window. Let yourself feel what it's like to be in that being's presence. Allow yourself to enjoy the good company.

3. Recognize how vulnerable this loved one is—just like you, subject to sickness, aging, and death. Also, this being wishes to be happy and free from suffering, just like you and every other living being. Repeat softly and gently, feeling the importance of your words:

    May you be safe.
    May you be peaceful.
    May you be healthy.
    May you live with ease.

    If you notice that your mind has wandered, return to the words and the image of the loved one you have in mind. Savor any warm feelings that may arise. Go slowly.

4. Add yourself to your circle of goodwill. Keep your hands over your heart and feel the warmth and gentle pressure of your hands (for just a moment or for the rest of the meditation), saying:

    May you and I be safe.
    May you and I be peaceful.
    May you and I be healthy.
    May you and I live with ease.

5. Visualize your whole body in your mind's eye, notice any stress or uneasiness that may be lingering within you, and offer kindness to yourself:

    May I be safe.
    May I be peaceful.
    May I be healthy.
    May I live with ease.

6. Take a few breaths and sit quietly in your own body, savoring the good-will and compassion that flows naturally from your own heart. Know that you can return to the phrases anytime you wish.

7. Gently open your eyes.

Source: Used with permission from Christopher Germer, *Mindful Self-Compassion* (www.mindfulselfcompassion.org), February 16, 2013.

C

Meditation on the Heart

The meditation on the heart is a heart rhythm meditation (HRM) that focuses on the breath and heartbeat, making the breath full, deep, rich, rhythmic, and balanced. Attention is focused on the heart as the center of the energetic system. This is a practice that energizes the body and moves the consciousness toward self-awareness and self-compassion.

1. Sit up straight and tall, so that your spine is straight, your posture is upright but relaxed, and your chest is open.

2. Pay attention to your breathing. Nearly all forms of meditation involve conscious breath. If this is as far as you go, then you will achieve great benefit. But at some point, you'll want to go further. You may also realize just how difficult it is to stay conscious of your breath, as your mind tends to wander to other things.

3. Adopt the point of view that it is your heart that breathes. Simply sit up straight, pay attention to your breath, and feel that your heart is breathing in and out. This is very powerful and will energize your heart beautifully. Yet there is more.

4. Make your breath balanced and rhythmic, so that the inhalation is the same length and intensity as the exhalation. The point of rhythmic breath is to even out the energetic imbalances that have their foundation in an uneven breath. If the inhalation is longer, the exhalation must be more intense to make up the same breath volume. Because the inhalation represents receiving and the exhalation represents giving, you can see how an imbalance in the breath can reverberate into every aspect of your life.

5. Make your breath very deep and full by engaging your abdominal muscles as you exhale and opening as much as you can on the inhale. Breathing fully is the key to a great source of energy. After you experience the power of full breath, you'll never want to return to a shallow breath.

6. Pay attention to your heartbeat. If you can't feel it, don't worry. Just keep trying. We know that about 50% of people who try don't feel it right away. Just keep paying attention, and it will come. Your heartbeat will get stronger and stronger the more you pay attention to it, and trying to feel it is a powerful way of paying attention.

7. Coordinate your breath and heartbeat by breathing in the same number of heartbeats that you breathe out—e.g., eight beats in, eight beats out.

8. Take a word or phrase that is sacred to you in some way and place the syllables of it on your heartbeat. For example, perhaps that word is *ocean*. This word has two syllables, which correspond nicely to the double-beat of the

heart, lub dub. Instead of counting, you simply say the word ocean to yourself as you breathe and pay attention to your heartbeat. Some prefer to place a sacred word or phrase on the breath rather than the heartbeat.

9. Now think of an infinite quality that you recognize in the word or phrase you are using. To continue with the example, think of the infinite energy, power, flexibility, and abundance of the ocean. Bring that energy into your own heart; recognize that these qualities are present in you as well, that you are as large as what you call upon.

10. Imagine merging yourself with your breath. Let the practice take over until there is no more self left, just the perfection of energy, power, flexibility, abundance—or whatever qualities you were focusing on. Let yourself be lost for a moment, eclipsed by the experience of the infinite within your heart.

Source: Excerpted and revised with permission from Asatar Bair, February 15, 2013 (www.iam-u.org/index.php/how-to-meditate-on-your-heart)

D

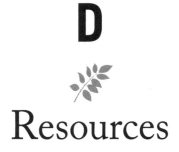

Resources

Programs in Whole-Person Caring

The Model of Whole-Person Caring

Address: 12592 Valley Vista Ln., Fresno, CA
93730
Phone: (559) 824-4702
Email: lucia@luciathornton.com
Website: www.luciathornton.com

Lucia Thornton offers consultation and educational programs on the model of whole-person caring and holistic nursing practice. A 2-day interprofessional program is available to individuals, health care and educational organizations, and communities to jump-start participants toward healthier and more wholesome ways of living and working. Facilitator training is also available for those wanting to create ongoing health and wellness programs in their organizations.

McGill University, Program in Whole-Person Care

Address:	Gerald Bronfman Centre, 546 Pine Ave. W., Montreal, Quebec, H2W 1S6
Phone:	(514) 398-2298
Fax:	(514) 398-5111
Email:	tom.hutchinson@mcgill.ca
Website:	www.mcgill.ca/wholepersoncare

The mission of the Program in Whole-Person Care is to transform Western medicine by synergizing the power of modern biomedicine with the potential for healing of every person who seeks the help of a health care practitioner. This objective is achieved by serving as champions for whole-person care at McGill and in the wider community through teaching, research, and translation of knowledge. The program offers workshops, seminars, videos, and an annual conference for health care professionals and all individuals interested in healing the whole person.

Professional Organizations for Healing and Wellness

American Holistic Health Association

Address:	P.O. Box 17400, Anaheim, CA 92817-7400
Phone:	(714) 779-6152
Email:	mail@ahha.org
Website:	www.ahha.org

The American Holistic Health Association (AHHA) is a free, impartial clearinghouse of wellness resources to help people become more active and confident in their health decisions. AHHA is endorsed by leading health care professionals worldwide. The AHHA website and blog offer a wide variety of both conventional and alternative self-help resources.

The American Holistic Medical Association

Address:	27629 Chagrin Blvd., Ste. 206, Woodmere, OH 44122
Phone:	(216) 292-6644
Fax:	(216) 292-6688
Email:	info@holisticmedicine.org
Website:	www.holisticmedicine.org

The American Holistic Medical Association (AHMA) was founded in 1978 by physicians to explore and advance holistic medical practice through annual conferences, publications, and member services. While the majority of members are MDs and DOs, members also include DCs, NDs, NPs, RNs, PAs, LACs, and MTs; practitioners of tradional Chinese medicine (TCM) and Ayurveda; and many others, strengthening the organization through its integrative diversity. AHMA distinguishes itself from other integrative-medicine associations in that it does not focus on any one modality or set of modalities and instead aligns itself with holistic medical principles. AHMA holds an annual conference and meeting, and it connects tens of thousands of people annually who seek integrative holistic care to AHMA members. A comprehensive listing of integrative medical centers can be found at the AHMA website (www.holisticmedicine.org/content.asp?pl=30&sl=2&contentid=7).

American Holistic Nurses Association

Address:	100 SE 9th St., Ste. 3A, Topeka, KS 66612-1213
Phone:	(800) 278-2462
	(785) 234-1712
Fax:	(785) 234-1713
Email:	info@ahna.org
Website:	www.ahna.org/

The American Holistic Nurses Association (AHNA) is a nonprofit membership association whose mission is to advance holistic nursing through community building, advocacy, research, and education. AHNA provides a supportive community, informative publications, continuing education, local networking opportunities, an annual conference, and support for research.

The Samueli Institute

Address:	1737 King St., Ste. 600, Alexandria, VA 22314
Phone:	(703) 299-4800
Fax:	(703) 535-6752
Email:	services@samueliinstitute.org
Website:	www.siib.org

The Samueli Institute is a nonprofit research organization supporting the scientific exploration of healing processes and their role in medicine, with the mission of transforming health care worldwide. The Samueli Institute facilitates activities in society that serve to align whole-person healing with science and action; create policies that promote wellness; link productivity and profit to health promotion; facilitate ways of learning, working, and playing that create health and community well-being; and inform a biomedical and health care system that heals as well as cures.

The Society for Scientific Exploration

Address: 151 Petaluma Blvd. S., #227, Petaluma, CA 94952
Phone: (415) 435-1604
Email: ericksoneditorial@gmail.com
Website: www.scientificexploration.org

The Society for Scientific Exploration (SSE) is a professional organization of scientists and scholars who study unusual and unexplained phenomena. Subjects often cross mainstream boundaries, such as consciousness, unidentified aerial phenomena, and alternative medicine, yet often have profound implications for human knowledge and technology. The SSE publishes a peer-reviewed journal, the *Journal of Scientific Exploration (JSE)*, and holds annual meetings in the United States and biennial meetings in Europe. Associate and student memberships are available to the public, and everyone is encouraged to attend meetings and participate with the society. A quarterly magazine, *EdgeScience* (www.scientificexploration.org/edgescience/), is offered free to the public.

Meditation Resources

Mindful Self Compassion

Address: 94 Pleasant St., Arlington, MA 02476-6533
Email: centerformsc@gmail.com
Website: www.centerformsc.org
www.mindfulselfcompassion.org

Christopher Germer, PhD, offers workshops internationally on mindfulness and self-compassion. Online courses, publications, and free meditation downloads can be accessed on the websites.

Self-Realization Fellowship

Address:	880 San Rafael Ave., Los Angeles, CA 90065
Phone:	(323) 225-2471
Fax:	(323) 225-5088
Website:	www.yogananda-srf.org

Founded in 1920 by Paramahansa Yogananda, author of *Autobiography of a Yogi*, this organization provides in-depth guidance in all aspects of physical, mental, and spiritual development that are centered around scientific methods of meditation. Home-study courses are available as well as formal and informal retreats and meditation gatherings in cities around the world and a worldwide prayer circle for healing.

Spirit Rock Meditation Center

Address:	P.O. Box 169, Woodacre, CA 94973
Phone:	(415) 488-0164
Website:	www.spiritrock.org

Founded by Jack Kornfield, this organization provides individuals, families, and children with information, classes, and retreats on mindfulness meditation.

University of Massachusetts Medical School

Address:	55 Lake Ave. N., Worcester, MA 01655
Phone:	(508) 856-2656
Email:	mindfulness@umassmed.edu
Website:	www.umassmed.edu/cfm

Established in 1995, the Center for Mindfulness in Medicine, Health Care, and Society emerged as an outgrowth of the Stress Reduction Clinic, founded by Dr. Jon Kabat-Zinn in 1979. In 2001, Dr. Saki Santorelli established the Oasis Institute of MBSR Professional Education and Training. In 2003, Dr. Santorelli established the annual international scientific conference on mindfulness. Today, the Center for Mindfulness in Medicine, Health Care, and Society continues to offer the 8-week MBSR program along with a variety of mindfulness programs for individuals, organizations, and communities ranging from half-day sessions to multiweek programs to certification to teach MBSR. In support of its programs, the Center for Mindfulness in Medicine, Health Care, and Society also offers educational materials to assist health care professionals, teachers, students, and laypeople to bring mind-body health and awareness into their lives.

Subtle Energy and Body-Based Therapies

Healing Touch International, Inc.

Address: 445 Union Blvd., Ste. 105, Lakewood, CO 80228
Phone: (303) 989-7982
Fax: (303) 980-8683
Website: www.healingtouchinternational.org

Healing Touch International is a nonprofit certification, education, and membership organization that serves healing touch providers, instructors, and the general public. The organization, established in 1996, certifies healing touch practitioners and instructors, coordinates healing touch research, assists integration of healing touch into health care settings, and promotes the work of healing touch around the world.

Healing Touch Program

Address: 20822 Cactus Loop, San Antonio, TX 78258
Phone: (210) 497-5529
Fax: (210) 497-8532
Email: info@healingtouchprogram.com
Website: www.healingtouchprogram.com

Healing Touch Program (HTP) is an educational program dedicated to offering classes in the energetic therapy modality of healing touch (HT) as well as providing support for healing touch students, practitioners, and instructors. HTP offers instructor credentialing along with continuing education units and is open to all nurses, massage therapists, body therapists, counselors, psychotherapists, physicians, and other allied health care professionals, as well as individuals who desire an in-depth understanding and practice of healing work using energy-based concepts and principles.

International Institute of Reflexology

Address: 5650 First Ave. N., P.O. Box 12642, St. Petersburg, FL 33710
Phone: (727) 343-4811
Fax: (727) 381-2807
Email: iir@reflexology-usa.net
Website: www.reflexology-usa.net

This membership and educational organization offers a certification program and advanced training in reflexology with classes held throughout the United States. The institute offers a variety of publications, charts, and references for the practice of reflexology.

The International Society for the Study of Subtle Energies and Energy Medicine (ISSSEEM)

Website: www.issseem.org

The International Society for the Study of Subtle Energies and Energy Medicine (ISSSEEM), organized in 1989, is an interdisciplinary organization for the study of the basic sciences and medical and therapeutic applications of subtle energies. ISSSEEM holds conferences and maintains an archive of the Subtle Energies and Energy Medicine Journal (SEEMJ) and Bridges magazine that is available online for public use. SEEMJ is a scholarly journal concerning consciousness, healing, and human potential addressing the study of subtle energies and informational systems interacting with the human psyche and physiology. The archives for the journal can be accessed at journals.sfu.ca/seemj/index.php/seemj. Bridges magazine presents articles, reports, and interviews with personal , clinical and experiential perspectives exploring ideas in the field of subtle energies, energy healing, and consciousness, and serves as a bridge between science and spirituality. Past issues of Bridges can be accessed at www.issseem.org/bridges-archive.cfm.

Jin Shin Jyutsu, Inc.

Address: 8719 E. San Alberto St., Scottsdale, AZ 85258
Phone: (480) 998-9331
Fax: (480) 998-9335
Email: info@jsjinc.com
Website: www.jsjinc.net

This organization provides information, publications, and a variety of courses on the practice and art of Jin Shin Jyutsu. Jin Shin Jyutsu is an ancient healing art that uses the gentle pressure of the hands to stimulate the energy flow within the body, restoring balance and harmony. Nursing CEUs are available for some of the classes.

Qigong Healing: The Chi Center

Address:	101 San Antonio Rd., Petaluma, CA 94952
Phone:	(707) 347-6489
Email:	admin@chicenter.com
Website:	www.chicenter.com

Founded by qigong master Ming Tong Gu, the Chi Center offers Web-based seminars, weekend programs, community healing events, teacher training, and an ongoing support system to provide sustainable healing practice for individuals and communities. The Chi Center's mission is to facilitate the integration of mind, body, and spirit by sharing the skill, knowledge, love, and energy of the ancient art and new science of wisdom-healing qigong.

Therapeutic Touch International Association, Inc.

Address:	P.O. Box 130, Delmar, NY, 12054
Phone:	(518) 325-1185
Fax:	(509) 693-3537
Email:	info@therapeutic-touch.org
Website:	www.therapeutic-touch.org

It is the mission of Therapeutic Touch International Association (TTIA) (formerly Nurse Healers–Professional Associates International, or NH-PAI) to lead, inspire, and advance excellence in therapeutic touch as a healing practice and way of life. The association serves as the central resource for information on therapeutic touch and participates in the ongoing development of therapeutic touch practice, teaching, credentialing, and research. The association promulgates standards for therapeutic touch education and practice; viewing the human body as a complex, dynamic whole; and healing as a process of restoring and promoting the integrity of body, mind, and spirit.

Naturopathic Medicine

Bastyr University

Address: 14500 Juanita Dr. N.E., Kenmore, WA 98028-4966
Phone: (425) 602-3000
Fax: (425) 823-6222
Website: www.bastyr.edu

Bastyr University is internationally recognized as a pioneer in natural medicine. Combining a science-based natural health curriculum with leading-edge research and clinical training, Bastyr University educates future leaders in fields such as naturopathic medicine, acupuncture and Oriental medicine, and whole-food nutrition. With campuses in Seattle and San Diego, the university now offers more than 17 accredited degree and certificate programs.

East-West Medicine

UCLA Center for East-West Medicine

Clinics

Address:	2336 Santa Monica Blvd., Ste. 301, Santa Monica, CA 90404
Phone:	(310) 998-9118
Address:	1250 La Venta Dr., Ste. 105, Westlake Village, CA 91361
Phone:	(855) Go 2 UCLA

Administrative Office

Address:	1033 Gayley Ave., Ste. 111, Los Angeles, CA 90024
Phone:	(310) 794-0712
Email:	cewm@mednet.ucla.edu
Website:	www.cewm.med.ucla.edu/

The purpose of the center is to develop a comprehensive system of care with emphasis on health promotion, disease prevention, treatment, and rehabilitation through the integrated practice of East-West medicine. The center offers clinical services and educational programs in integrative medicine. A 6-week summer course for all health professionals and students provides an introduction to integrative health care, particularly the therapeutic approaches originating from TCM (exploreim.ucla.edu/events/med-180-summer-course/). A website of resources exclusively about integrative medicine can be found here: exploreim.ucla.edu/.

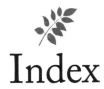

Index

J–K

I

L

O

P

W–X

Y–Z